Also by William H. Parker, M.D., and Rachel Parker

A Gynecologist's Second Opinion: The Questions and Answers You Need to Take Care of Your Health

the INCONTINENCE SOLUTION

ANSWERS FOR WOMEN OF ALL AGES

William H. Parker, M.D.
Amy E. Rosenman, M.D.
Rachel Parker

A FIRESIDE BOOK
PUBLISHED BY SIMON & SCHUSTER
New York   London   Toronto   Sydney   Singapore

Note to the reader: This book has been written to provide educational material for women and is not intended as a substitute for medical care from a doctor or other health professionals. Medicine is an evolving field, and new research and ideas may lead to changes in some of the concepts presented here. The reader should consult her doctor or other health professional concerning any health matters.

FIRESIDE
Rockefeller Center
1230 Avenue of the Americas
New York, NY 10020

FIRESIDE and colophon are registered trademarks
of Simon & Schuster, Inc.

For information about special discounts for bulk purchases,
please contact Simon & Schuster Special Sales:
1-800-456-6798 or business@simonandschuster.com

Designed by Christine Weathersbee
Line illustrations by Peggy Firth, medical illustrator
Manufactured in the United States of America

10 9 8 7 6 5 4 3 2 1

Library of Congress Cataloging-in-Publication Data

Parker, William H., M.D.
    The incontinence solution : answers for women of all ages /
William H. Parker, Amy E. Rosenman, Rachel L. Parker.
        p.   cm.
    "A Fireside book."
    Includes bibliographical references and index.
    1. Urinary incontinence.   2. Urinary incontinence—Treatment.
3. Women—Diseases—Treatment.   I. Rosenman, Amy E., 1951–
II. Parker, Rachel L.   III. Title.

RC921 .I5 P375 2002
616.6'2—dc21   2002016372

ISBN 0-7432-1587-7

*To Aaron, Evan, and Brian, sons we love beyond words;
and to our parents, Renee, Sid, Esther, and Stanley
(in loving memory), for loving support.*
                              —William H. Parker, Rachel Parker

*To Rachel and Matthew, my children, who have taught me
more than I could possibly teach them; and to Bill Rogers,
my husband, for his never-ending support.*
                              —Amy E. Rosenman

Many people helped during the writing of this book, and we are thankful to them. We are enormously grateful to our agent, Arielle Eckstut, for her lucid advice and abundant enthusiasm for this project; and to our editor, Lisa Considine, for her suggestions, support, and careful guidance to its completion. Peggy Firth, our medical illustrator, once again provided clear, understandable diagrams and was a pleasure to work with. We also thank William Rogers Photography for the excellent photographs he provided.

A number of our teachers, colleagues, and friends took the time to review the manuscript and offer their special expertise: Dr. Alfred Bent, head of the Division of Urogynecology and Reconstructive Pelvic Surgery, Greater Baltimore Medical Center, Baltimore, Maryland; Dr. Narender Bhatia, head of the Division of Urogynecology and Reconstructive Pelvic Surgery, Harbor–UCLA Hospital, Torrance, California; Dr. Mickey Karram, director of Urogynecology at Good Samaritan Hospital, Cincinnati, Ohio; Dr. C. Y. Lui, director, Chattanooga Woman's Laser Surgery Center, Chattanooga, Tennessee; Dr. Peggy Norton, division chief, Department of Urogynecology and Reconstructive Pelvic Surgery, University of Utah, Salt Lake City, Utah; Dr. Donald Ostergard, director of Division of Urogynecology, University of California, Irvine, California; Dr. W. Conrad Sweeting, Urogynecology Section, Kaiser Medical Center, San Francisco, California; Dr. Bob Shull, director, Section of Urogynecology and Reconstructive Pelvic Surgery, Temple, Texas; Dr. Joshua Golden, director, Human Sexuality Program, UCLA School of Medicine, Westwood, California; Dr. Beth Meyerowitz,

Department of Psychology, University of Southern California, Los Angeles, California. We thank them all for their invaluable help.

We would like to thank our partner, Ingrid Rodi, M.D., for her intelligence and her support. We would also like to thank all of our teachers over the years who have given freely of their time and knowledge; and all of our patients, who have allowed us to care for them and who have taught us so much.

CONTENTS

Introduction

Today there are approximately 25 million Americans suffering from an ailment that many are unwilling to disclose. Even more poignant, many of those 25 million could be cured fairly quickly. So why won't they talk about incontinence? We seem to be busy talking about practically everything else. Topics once considered taboo now entertain millions of television viewers every day. We watch people—famous people, no less—discussing family troubles, drug and alcohol abuse, even impotence. But the indignity of incontinence remains in the closet.

The majority of the silent sufferers are women. While incontinence is usually considered a problem only of the elderly, the truth is that more than 50 percent of healthy women between the ages of forty-two and fifty have some degree of incontinence—30 percent of these younger women on a regular basis! And while many of these women make significant adjustments in their lifestyle to hide the problem, the majority of women with incontinence do not talk to their doctors or even their best friends about it. A staggering 90 percent of all women with incontinence do not seek any medical care for this problem.

Perhaps these women think that if they have incontinence at a young age, it must be their own fault. Some believe they didn't do enough Kegel exercises after having children, or that they lifted too many heavy objects. Older women erroneously believe that loss of urine is one of those things that happens "naturally" as they age. It is not. Although incontinence is more common in women over age sixty, the majority of elderly women are not incontinent.

Older women with incontinence may have very different concerns than do their younger counterparts. Older women often fear that their incontinence will lead to rejection by family members. Some worry that incontinence will mean a certain move to a nursing home. For women of all ages, keeping the problem a secret helps maintain a false sense of normalcy. Embarrassment is the biggest obstacle to seeking appropriate care for incontinence.

Doctors and other health care providers often make the problem worse by ignoring it. Most doctors and health care professionals don't ask patients about incontinence for any number of reasons—perhaps because they lack the time or knowledge to treat it properly, perhaps because the topic makes them uncomfortable too. The National Institutes of Health (NIH) realized that undiagnosed and untreated incontinence was an enormous medical problem and in 1996 developed guidelines for doctors, stressing the importance of asking patients about it. The fact that the federal government's health agency recognized that doctors often ignore this major health care issue underscores the scope of the problem. Doctors and patients are in need of education on the causes and treatment options for this all-too-common problem.

Incontinence deserves the same attention you would give to other medical conditions, such as high blood pressure or diabetes. Incontinence is a medical problem. It is not the result of poor manners, bad behavior, or faulty upbringing. Fixing the problem will help end the embarrassment. You are never too old or too young to seek care for this troubling problem. What most silent, suffering women don't realize is that there is a wide range of treatments for incontinence problems, many of which don't involve surgery.

Untreated incontinence can lead to other health problems. Incontinence, urgency, and frequency of urination often disturb sleep and lead to chronic fatigue and grumpiness. In order to avoid embarrassing accidents, many women with incontinence withdraw from physical activity, effectively chipping away at one of the cornerstones of good health. For starters, regular exercise decreases the risk of heart disease, a major killer of women today. Staying active also aids in weight control and the maintenance of normal blood pressure and keeps bones strong and healthy. It plays a role in mental health too, decreasing depression and anxiety by increasing the level of beneficial endorphins in the brain that create a sense of well-being.

Incontinent women also report withdrawing from social situations, which can lead to isolation and depression. The sobering bottom line is that a woman who decides to grin and bear incontinence may soon find every aspect of her life diminished.

Despite the enormity of this problem, there is very little information available for women to help them understand the causes and, more important, the available treatments for incontinence. In this book we'll take a look at current medical thinking and explain state-of-the-art remedies. New techniques in the fields of gynecology and urology now enable us to help more and more women with bladder problems. No woman should simply endure them.

If Oprah Winfrey knew that 20 million women were suffering silently from incontinence, do you think she would ignore them? The media have been silent on this issue for far too long, and as a result many women feel alone and discouraged from getting help. We hope to break that silence with this book.

the
INCONTINENCE
SOLUTION

CHAPTER 1

Defining Incontinence

WHAT IS INCONTINENCE?

Incontinence is the uncontrollable loss of enough urine to cause social or sanitary difficulties. When we study the body and look at how we control urination, we know that an infant does not have the proper connections between its brain and bladder to be able to control the bladder. We also know that as the brain develops, young children can be taught to control when and where they empty their bladders. This learned control is then maintained, usually without much thought, throughout adulthood. To a child or an adult, any loss of bladder control feels like a return to infancy and can be an embarrassment and a source of terrible discomfort.

Incontinence can be a significant problem for young, middle-aged, and older women. Life with incontinence, even mild incontinence, can become very stressful as it threatens self-image, body image, and self-esteem. Concerns about having to deal with incontinence may hinder career opportunities for women in the workforce. The embarrassing loss of self-control makes a woman feel old and helpless. Outings for shopping and recreation may be planned around the availability of bathrooms. Travel to new places becomes difficult. Having a change of clothes handy and worrying about odor are constant concerns. Worst of all, women suffering from incontinence may stop some of the activities they enjoy altogether; they may avoid getting together with friends or family and having sexual contact altogether. Understandably, they may feel depressed.

Many people consider adult incontinence a natural part of aging. It is not! The vast majority of older women do not have incontinence. Most people are not aware that young women can also have incontinence. Since incontinence is so frequently associated with aging, younger women are even less likely to talk about it or seek treatment. The good news is that there are now many ways to treat women of all ages who have incontinence.

IS ALL INCONTINENCE THE SAME?

Incontinence is a symptom—the loss of urine. The two most common types of incontinence are loss of urine with laughing, coughing, or sneezing, called *stress incontinence,* and loss of urine preceded by a strong urge to go, called *urge incontinence* or *overactive bladder.* Sometimes a woman has both types of incontinence at the same time. This combination of types of incontinence is called *mixed incontinence.* Different types of incontinence have different causes, and different treatments solve each type. The first step toward ending incontinence is for your doctor to determine which type of incontinence you have. This begins with your answering questions about your symptoms. Following that, a number of simple tests are performed to help pinpoint the nature of the problem, which we will discuss in Chapter 3. But first, it will be helpful to understand what the possible types of incontinence are. The chart below gives brief definitions of the types of incontinence. More detailed explanations follow.

TYPES OF INCONTINENCE

STRESS incontinence:	Urine loss with some type of physical stress to the body such as with a cough, sneeze, physical activity, or laughing.
URGE incontinence:	Urine loss preceded by a sense of needing to urinate before reaching the bathroom.
MIXED incontinence:	Urine loss with features of both stress and urge.
OVERFLOW incontinence:	Urine loss occurring when the bladder is full but the bladder does not contract properly to push the urine out. The urine then trickles out of the overfull bladder.
TOTAL incontinence:	The constant loss of urine.

WHAT HAPPENS WHEN A LAUGH, COUGH, OR SNEEZE CAUSES LEAKING?

You may have noticed that sometimes a loss of urine occurs as a result of a cough, sneeze, laugh, or vigorous exercise. Many women with this problem, known as stress incontinence, may begin limiting their own activities for just this reason. However, coughing, sneezing, and even laughing are often unavoidable. We need to laugh and exercise (and cough and sneeze) to live life to its fullest. Understanding stress incontinence is the first step toward finding a solution.

Stress incontinence got its name because the pressure or strain from a laugh or cough results in a loss of urine. The bladder and urethra are normally held firmly in place by muscles and connect-

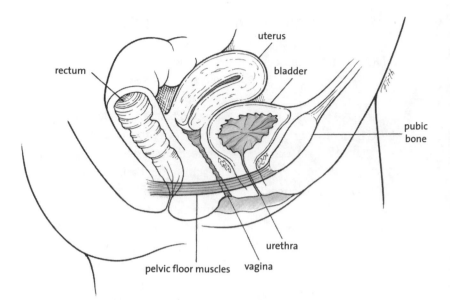

Figure 1-1: NORMAL PELVIC ORGANS AND MUSCLES

ing tissue in the pelvis (Figure 1-1). When you cough, the pressure inside your abdomen increases, and the pressure pushes on your bladder and urethra. If the supporting pelvic muscles or connecting tissues have been damaged or weakened, they may not be able to withstand the force of the cough. The pressure then forces the urethra to open, and urine leaks out (Figure 1-2). Many activities that you ordinarily wouldn't even think about can cause increased pressure in the abdomen and the bladder. Coughing, straining to lift a heavy piece of luggage, aerobic exercise, or even a hiccup can challenge a woman with this problem.

WHAT CAUSES STRESS INCONTINENCE?

As we discuss in Chapter 4, pregnancy and childbirth can damage the pelvic ligaments that anchor the uterus and bladder to the bones of the pelvis. The muscles that support the bladder work dif-

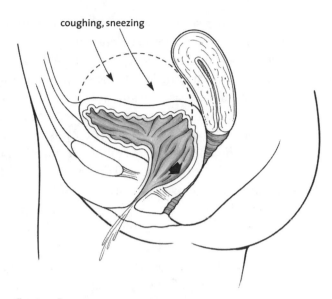

Figure 1-2: STRESS INCONTINENCE

ferently from most other muscles. Other muscles in your body usually relax until you ask them to do something for you, such as lifting a fork or bending at the waist. However, the pelvic muscles are always contracted so that they can continually hold up the bladder, uterus, and intestines. If these muscles, and the connecting tissue that attaches the muscles to the pelvic bones, are stretched or damaged, as may happen during childbirth, they become less effective at holding things up. The urethra may then be pushed out of position by a cough, sneeze, or strenuous activity because the muscle support cannot withstand the extra pressure.

The nerves sending messages from the brain to the pelvic muscles may also be altered due to childbirth. In the birth canal, the baby's head puts pressure on these nerves. Prolonged pressure, or undue pressure because of the size of the baby's head, may damage these nerves so they cannot send proper signals to the supporting muscles. As a result, the muscles may not be able to hold the bladder up.

Other factors may also cause increased pressure on the pelvic organs that probably contributes to incontinence. A family history of incontinence may be an important factor since the amount and strength of the collagen that makes up the supporting tissue is inherited. Smoking can decrease the amount of oxygen the muscles and ligaments get and thereby lead to weakened tissues. In addition, smokers often cough, and every cough pushes against the bladder and pelvic ligaments and, over time, may weaken them. If a woman is overweight, extra pressure is added to an already weakened system and may aggravate the problem of leakage. Chronic constipation, which causes straining to pass a bowel movement, also increases the abdominal pressure and can weaken the support of the bladder and pelvic organs.

In some women, the hormonal changes that occur with menopause can cause thinning of the tissues and blood vessels of the urethra. Try to visualize the urethra as a tube—if you were to cut across it, the cross section would look like a doughnut. With declining estrogen levels, the walls of this tube shrink, resulting in a larger hole. The larger the opening, the more difficult it is for the muscles to seal. If the urethra is not closed, urine can leak out (Figure 1-3).

Any one or more of these factors—stretched pelvic muscles, excess body weight, damaged nerves, or thinning of the urethra—may lead to stress incontinence. As you will see in later chapters, treatment for this type of incontinence involves strengthening the pelvic muscles or repairing the supporting tissues to the bladder and urethra.

WHAT IF YOU HAVE THE URGE TO URINATE FREQUENTLY?

Urgency is the sense that you have to urinate right now. When you gotta go, you gotta go. The constant urge to empty the bladder and

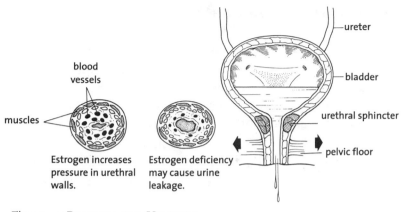

Figure 1-3: BLADDER AND URETHRA

all those trips to the bathroom can be disabling to many women. They do not necessarily leak urine, but their lives are nevertheless taken over by their bladder problems. Urgency is basically the result of the bladder misbehaving, of the bladder being overactive. In fact, the term *overactive bladder* is now frequently used instead of urgency. Instead of quietly collecting urine, the bladder is constantly making a nuisance of itself. This is perceived as everpresent bladder pressure. The bladder feels as if it is always full, but in fact most trips to the toilet produce no more than a few ounces of urine. Some women may note urgency during the night that wakes them repeatedly.

Urgency and frequency are frustrating problems. Many women suffer in silence because they do not realize that, thankfully, there are many solutions to their problem. These include taking prescription medication, learning to urinate on a schedule, and doing muscle exercises that can help reduce spasms. Simple dietary changes may also help reduce frequency and urgency. These nonsurgical treatments and others are fully discussed in Chapter 5.

HOW COMMON IS URGENCY?

Urgency is one area where age does seem to make a difference. About 6 percent of women under forty have symptoms of urgency, and about 10 percent of women have this symptom prior to menopause. By the time women reach their late fifties and early sixties, about 40 percent will have urgency. And by the time women reach their eighties, nearly 80 percent have this problem. About 40 percent of women who develop urgency also have urge incontinence, meaning urgency to the degree that they may actually lose urine.

WHAT CAUSES A STRONG URGE TO URINATE?

The most common temporary cause of having a strong urge to urinate is a bladder infection. The infection causes an irritation of the bladder lining that leads to spasms of the bladder muscle. However, the bladder irritation and urgency go away once the infection is treated with antibiotics. Only rarely does a bladder infection lead to such severe urgency that incontinence results. If treated, these infections have no permanent effect on your bladder.

Unlike with stress incontinence, childbirth does not appear to play any role in the development of urgency. Most women's urgency problems are not easily explained. A number of theories suggest what the causes might be, but none have been proven. Some researchers focus on the nerve signals to the bladder. They suggest that some women may have a mild, probably age-related, change in the nerves or the chemical signals between the nerves that leads to overactivity of the bladder. Some propose that the problem is rooted in the muscle cells of the bladder itself, which may be overactive. This theory is supported by the fact that about 50 percent of women with urge incontinence also have a similar problem with their intestines called irritable bowel syndrome. The overactivity of the muscle cells in the intestines that occurs with irritable bowel syndrome leads to abdominal cramping.

Some women have overactivity of the bladder from causes that are easier to establish. Women who have had multiple surgeries to correct incontinence are at a slightly higher risk of developing urgency and urge incontinence. In these women, the bladder nerves may be injured after being pulled, stretched, or even cut at the time of surgery. In others, previous surgery may have caused scar tissue to block the flow of urine out of the bladder. The bladder then needs to work harder to get the urine out past the scar tissue, and the overworked bladder muscle may function poorly.

Another condition associated with bothersome frequency and urgency is called *interstitial cystitis*, or IC. IC may also be associated with recurrent discomfort or pain in both the bladder and the nearby pelvic area. Interstitial cystitis is fully discussed in Chapter 7.

Conditions affecting the nervous system, such as Parkinson's disease, multiple sclerosis, Alzheimer's disease, or stroke, may also cause urge incontinence. Other rare conditions such as benign polyps or stone formation in the bladder can also lead to urgency and incontinence. These problems can easily be evaluated with a cystoscope, a small telescope that allows the doctor to look into the bladder. This office procedure, called a cystoscopy, takes only a few minutes. Prior to insertion of the cystoscope, a topical anesthetic in a gel form is inserted into the urethra in order to relieve discomfort. With the cystoscope, we can see irritation from interstitial cystitis or the presence of a bladder stone, bladder cancer, or overgrown bladder lining cells that form polyps.

WHAT IF THERE'S A STRONG URGE TO URINATE AND THEN YOU LOSE CONTROL?

Normally you make a conscious decision about when to empty your bladder. When you get the feeling that your bladder is full, you control the urge to urinate and make it to the bathroom in time. However, some women have an overactive bladder that tries to empty on its own, often without much warning. If you feel a bladder contraction that causes such a strong sense of urgency that you cannot control it, you may lose urine before you can get to the bathroom. This is called *urge incontinence*. The causes of this problem are similar to those described for urgency.

Some women may have urge incontinence when they put their hands in running water or hear water running. Some note urge incontinence when they change position rapidly, such as when they get up quickly from a chair. Others get urge incontinence when they return home with a full bladder, park the car, rush to the front door, and put the key in the door. The anticipation of relief triggers a bladder spasm. This is so common it has a name, "key-in-the-door incontinence." Women with urge incontinence report that it affects the quality of their lives more than do women who have stress incontinence, depression, or even diabetes. Urge incontinence often results in a larger amount of lost urine than stress incontinence and is often unpredictable. While you may be able to brace yourself when you are about to laugh or cough and prevent loss of urine from stress incontinence, there is little warning with urge incontinence. By the time you realize what is happening, it is too late. Hence, women with this problem are often subject to embarrassing accidents.

This is no small problem. The unpredictability often causes women to stay at home near a bathroom or to limit their activities to places where a bathroom will immediately be available. They may dress in dark colors that hide wetness. Fear of odor or loss of urine during intercourse may lead to avoidance of intimacy. This often leads to isolation and depression. Urge incontinence may occur at night, resulting in a wet bed that needs to be changed. Disturbed sleep and the resulting fatigue are common in women with this problem. Women with urge incontinence feel terrible about their condition but often delay seeing a doctor because they are depressed and feel helpless. These women are not aware of the available treatments, all *nonsurgical,* that are now used to help women with urge incontinence. A discussion of these treatments can be found in Chapter 5.

WHAT CAN CAUSE LEAKAGE
WITH EVEN MINOR ACTIVITY?

Some women have very frequent leakage. They often leak when their bladders are full, but they may also leak when their bladders are nearly empty. They may leak when they cough or sneeze, but sometimes they also note leakage even when they are lying down. These symptoms may result from a condition called *intrinsic sphincter deficiency,* or ISD. Women with this problem are often understandably miserable.

Although this is a relatively rare problem, it has a number of possible causes. The problem exists in the urethral sphincter, the muscles and soft tissue that surround the urethra and hold the urine in the bladder (Figure 1-4). The muscles are normally squeezed closed, continuously shutting off the flow of urine. The urethra, which is shaped like a tube, is lined with soft, cushioning tissue that helps to form a watertight seal. When you laugh or sneeze, the muscles around the urethra resist the added pressure. The muscles are supposed to relax only when you are ready to urinate.

However, prior injury to the muscles or soft tissues can weaken the watertight seal and may allow urine to leak out (Figure 1-5). This type of incontinence is called intrinsic sphincter deficiency because it is the watertight seal (the sphincter) that is not functioning properly (is deficient). One cause of this problem, ironically enough, is the result of previous surgery for incontinence. The healing process following surgery around the bladder and urethra may sometimes lead to scar tissue, which is much less supple than normal tissue. In rare cases, excessive scar tissue may be formed.

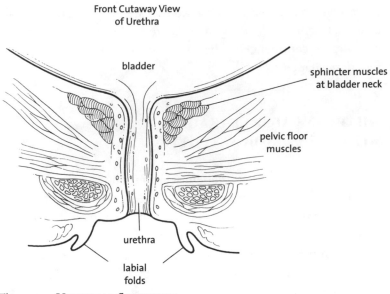

Figure 1-4: URETHRAL SPHINCTER

This can pull on the urethra and actually hold it open, allowing urine to leak out. In addition, the small nerves that carry signals to the urethra are not visible and may be inadvertently stretched or cut during surgery. Formation of scar tissue is not the result of poor surgical skills on the part of your doctor, but rather an unusual and unfortunate consequence of the body's healing process.

Another cause of this type of incontinence is radiation treatment for cancer. Radiation applied to the pelvic area can damage small blood vessels in the area, reducing the blood flow. Over time, often many years later, the radiation damage to the urethra can lead to thinning of the cushioning tissue that forms the watertight seal. As a result, the urethra does not close entirely, and incontinence is the result.

Age also appears to play a role in the development of ISD. As you age, the elasticity of the tissues decreases, and the watertight seal may not close off entirely. This type of very troubling inconti-

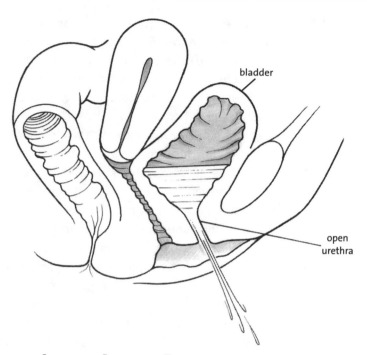

Figure 1-5: INTRINSIC SPHINCTER DEFICIENCY

nence probably results from a combination of aging, previous surgery, and radiation that eventually is significant enough to cause incontinence. The good news is that there are now a number of ways to help correct ISD (see Chapter 6).

Alice's Story

Tiny, quiet Alice came in to our office accompanied by her dutiful but frustrated son Dennis. At ninety-seven years of age, Alice was blessed with a relatively sound body and a sound mind. Her bladder, however, was no blessing to her. Ordinarily, Alice spent half the year in Los Angeles with Dennis and his family. For the other half of the year, she always traveled up to Oregon and stayed with her daughter Diane and her family. Winter and spring in Los Angeles, summer and fall in Oregon had been her routine for almost twenty years. This year, however, Alice would not leave her son's house for even an hour due to severe, constant loss of urine.

In her quiet way she made it clear that she had no intention of going to Oregon in this condition. Being wet all the time was naturally making her unhappy. The entire family was in an uproar, alternately worried about "this deterioration" and frustrated about her stubbornness. The seasonal routine was comfortable, and everyone was upset and fearful that it was over forever. This year had an extra significance since Alice's great-granddaughter Laurel was planning to be married in a great big June wedding, wearing lace from the bridal veil Alice herself had been married in seventy-six years before. During the months of planning, everyone was keeping their fingers crossed that great-grandma Alice would be there for the big day. As Dennis said, "It doesn't seem fair that after all she's been through in ninety-seven years, it comes down to wetting her pants." The big question in everyone's mind was "What can you do for a ninety-seven-year-old?"

Surgery as a solution to her incontinence seemed risky at her age. Nor did she want to put up with any recovery period, no matter how short. With a tremble in her chin, Alice said she knew that nothing could be done and she would just have to miss the wedding. But, as Dennis pointed out, the wedding was only a small part of the problem. Alice was now no longer willing to leave the house, and she was irritable and unhappy all the time. She had come today partly to get Dennis off her back, but now that she was in the office, she plaintively asked, "Is there any hope for me, doctor?"

We fully evaluated Alice with a complete history and physical. She was in remarkably good physical condition for her age. Her examination showed that there was some mild bulging of the bladder into the vagina. A complete evaluation, called urodynamic testing, showed that as we filled her bladder with fluid, it began to have spasms (overactivity) that led to urine leakage. The test also found that she had a very weak bladder sphincter. In thinking about the whole situation, we decided that collagen injections into the urethra would be the best bet for her. This procedure would help close off the urethral sphincter and could be performed under mild sedation in the hospital. She could get back home the same day, and the recovery would be painless and would last only a day. This solution would do nothing for the bulging bladder or its overactivity, but it would afford her extended periods of dryness each day. Alice and Dennis eagerly leapt at this "good enough" solution, and we proceeded with the collagen. Between her good physical health and her positive attitude, Alice recuperated quickly and was thrilled with the results. She still had some problems with the overactive bladder, but they were manageable. Within a few days she was taking an outing every day and was busy planning for the summer. She wore a pad for insurance and would need to have another collagen injection in a few months, but at her age she wasn't going to concern herself with that. In early June, Alice happily went off to Oregon, eagerly anticipating Laurel's wedding day.

WHAT IF YOU LEAK URINE ALL THE TIME?

In rare cases, women will note that they lose small amounts of urine all the time. Many of these women have no sensation that they are losing urine. Some note that when they try to urinate, the stream is weak or they only dribble. Pressing on the bladder or straining may be necessary in order to pass urine. This type of incontinence, called *overflow incontinence,* can be caused by a partial blockage of the flow of urine out of the bladder.

How can a blockage lead to the loss of urine? The blockage prevents you from fully emptying your bladder. As your kidneys make more urine, the bladder fills to capacity. Since the extra urine has nowhere to go, it pushes the watertight seal in the urethra open and urine trickles out, like water going over a dam. Women with this problem may also have frequent bladder infections because the trapped urine becomes a reservoir for bacteria that can multiply and cause an infection. Though a rare condition in women, overflow incontinence is much more common in older men. As men age, they often suffer from enlargement of the prostate gland. The prostate blocks the flow of urine out of the bladder, and the result is a constant trickle of urine.

WHAT CAN CAUSE YOU TO LEAK ALL THE TIME?

This is a rare condition, but there are a number of possible causes. Anything that blocks the urethra can lead to this condition. If the bladder drops (called cystocele or prolapse) and kinks the urethra, the kinking can prevent you from fully emptying your bladder. You may feel that your bladder is quite full, but as you attempt to urinate, only a small amount of urine is passed, and you do not feel empty. When your bladder fills to capacity, any additional urine leaks out, resulting in overflow incontinence. If kinking of the urethra is the problem, straightening out the bladder with a pessary or surgery will allow the bladder to empty properly and the problem will resolve.

In younger women, a contraceptive diaphragm can press on the urethra, making it difficult to empty the bladder with the diaphragm in place. Of course, if you remove the diaphragm, the blockage will be relieved and the problem will be fixed. Women who use a pessary may rarely notice a similar problem. On very rare occasions, a bladder infection makes urination so painful that you may hold urine in to avoid the pain. A herpes infection that occurs near the urethra can cause swelling and block the flow of urine. Over time the urine builds up until it dribbles out. These are just temporary situations that fade when the infections resolve.

Overflow incontinence is sometimes caused by an injury to the nerves that go to the bladder. This might be a temporary but severe injury to your back that puts pressure on the spinal cord or a permanent injury that might be the result of a serious accident that results in paralysis. Diseases that can affect the bladder nerves, such as multiple sclerosis, diabetes, or alcoholism, can interfere with the nerve signals to the bladder. If the proper messages cannot get from the brain to the bladder, the bladder cannot contract properly, and urine fills the bladder to the point of overflow.

Some medications can affect the nerve signals to the bladder. Though uncommon, medications such as anticonvulsants, antidepressants, or drugs for heart conditions, allergic conditions, or chemotherapy may sometimes lead to this type of incontinence. For this reason, it is a good idea to bring a list of your medications to the doctor when you are being treated for incontinence.

Another type of constant leaking occurs when the urethral muscle, the sphincter, doesn't *ever* close completely. This type of incontinence is called *total incontinence*. This is a very rare problem, sometimes related to an injury to the sphincter during childbirth or from previous surgery near the bladder. One more very rare cause of total incontinence is a fistula, a hole in the bladder that drains into the vagina. This problem can result from a difficult childbirth in which the vagina and bladder are torn, or it may result from an operation near the bladder, vagina, or uterus.

Although this sounds as though total incontinence may be caused by any number of things, it is actually very rare. Treatment for this condition is available using medications and, in some cases, surgery.

CHAPTER 2

How the Bladder Normally Works

WHERE DOES THE WATER GO?

Most of us have heard that water makes up 65 percent of the body and is vital to our survival. While we can live without food for a month, we can live without water for only a week! Maybe that's how the expression "dying of thirst" came about. We need water to dilute the nutrients in our food and to help carry energy all over our bodies. Water is necessary for the biochemical reactions that our cells use to function, grow and repair themselves. How does your body process the water and remove what's not needed? Let's follow a molecule of water on its path from your mouth all the way through your body.

We'll start with a cool glass of iced tea (mostly water) that you might drink at lunch on a hot summer day. As you swallow, the tea washes down your esophagus into your stomach. Your stomach starts the process of digestion, breaking food into smaller and smaller units that can easily be absorbed into the bloodstream to provide energy. The iced tea mixes with the food you have eaten, and after a few hours the contents of your stomach pass into the small intestines, which take up most of the area of your abdomen.

The nutrients from food, along with some water from the tea, are absorbed by the cells of the small intestines and passed into the bloodstream. Most of the remaining water is absorbed by the cells in the large intestines and passed into the bloodstream.

Once water gets into your bloodstream, it performs a number of essential tasks. It bathes the cells that make up your blood. New supplies of water replace any lost as a result of sweating. In addition, water is taken up by the cells to be used for the complex process of turning nutrients into energy. Last, water helps remove waste and toxins from the body. These wastes, which are mostly nitrogen compounds formed as by-products of the cells' energy use, are filtered out of the blood by the kidneys, which reabsorb most of the water and send it back into the bloodstream, preventing dehydration. The mixture of water and toxins, what we know as urine, collects in the center of the kidneys and then passes down through the ureters, small muscular tubes connecting to the bladder. When the bladder becomes full, your brain signals that you need to find a bathroom. Once you get to a bathroom, you relax the muscles holding the urine in. This voluntary relaxation of the muscles triggers a reflex contraction of the bladder muscle, and the urine, produced from that glass of iced tea you had for lunch, passes from your body. More detail about the normal workings of the bladder and kidneys follows.

WHAT IS THE BLADDER SUPPOSED TO DO?

The bladder has two basic functions. First, it stores the urine from the kidneys. The bladder fills up without any intentional thought on your part. Most women first sense urine in the bladder when there are about 4 ounces collected. As the bladder fills and stretches, the bladder nerves carry messages to the brain that it is time to find a bathroom. This usually happens when there are about 10 ounces in the bladder. All this is accomplished while the bladder painlessly expands and collects urine. At the point when the bladder is entirely full, containing about 15 to 20 ounces, you will feel uncomfortable and in need of relief, and will want to find a bathroom quickly.

The bladder's second function, releasing stored urine, is usually a conscious, voluntary act. When you get to the bathroom, you relax the muscle near the opening of the bladder, called the sphincter. At the same time that the sphincter relaxes, a reflex signal from the brain causes the bladder muscle to contract, and the urine is pushed out. The coordination of this system that keeps us dry is complicated, but we do all this with barely a thought. We learn this control when we are children, and it becomes second nature to us. The problem of incontinence arises when urine leaks out when we don't want it to.

HOW OFTEN SHOULD YOU NEED TO GO TO THE BATHROOM?

Most women who drink a normal amount of fluids will need to go to the bathroom about every three to four hours, or about six to eight times a day. Bladder infections can make you feel the need to go more often, as can an overactive bladder, a condition called interstitial cystitis, or an unusually small bladder. Also, the more fluids you drink, the more often you need to go.

HOW MUCH URINE SHOULD YOU PASS?

Most women first sense that they need to get to a bathroom when their bladder contains about 10 ounces of urine. Since the bladder can't hold much more than about 15 ounces, most women pass between 10 and 15 ounces of urine each time they urinate.

IS IT NORMAL TO GET UP AT NIGHT
TO GO TO THE BATHROOM?

It is normal to get up once or even twice in the middle of the night to urinate. If you are drinking a lot of fluids, drinking fluids late at night, or drinking caffeine or alcohol at night, you will probably have to get up more often for relief. Some women, especially older women with weaker hearts, retain fluid during the day and may notice swelling in their feet by evening. Gravity keeps this fluid in the feet and ankles, but once they lie down at night the fluid is free to move back into the bloodstream and is then pumped out by the kidneys. If this is the case, you will need to get up more often during the night to urinate. An overactive bladder (as discussed in Chapter 1) also creates the need to get up at night, even though the amount urinated is usually small.

IS LEAKING NORMAL?

If all the parts of the bladder are working properly, you should not leak any urine. That having been said, it is not unusual for women to occasionally leak a little urine during very heavy lifting, when they have a bad cough, or during very strenuous exercise. Some women notice that they leak when they hear running water or because they felt an urge to go and are on their way to the bathroom. This is usually a sign of an overactive bladder. If these leaking episodes persist or are bothersome in any way, you should consider evaluation by your physician.

IS BULGING OR DROPPING OF THE
BLADDER OR RECTUM NORMAL?

After childbirth, it is not unusual to have some bulging of the bladder or rectum into the vagina. This often goes away within a few months after delivery. However, for some women the bulging persists. As a woman ages, the supporting tissues in the pelvis may weaken, and the bulging may get more noticeable or bothersome. While bulging (prolapse) is not normal, it is common and not a danger to your health. Prolapse needs to be treated only if it bothers you. This is a quality-of-life decision, not a medical or health issue.

WHAT DO THE KIDNEYS DO?

The urinary system is made up of two kidneys, two ureters, and the bladder. The kidneys lie inside your abdominal cavity, toward your back, one on each side of and just below the level of your shoulder blades (Figure 2-1). Each kidney is about the size of your fist. Vital to the body, the kidneys filter waste and toxins out of the blood. They filter about 50 gallons of blood each and every day. Accomplishing this filtering process requires an amazing and complicated arrangement of small tubes within the kidney that are specially designed to remove waste while allowing water, proteins, and glucose to be reabsorbed and rejoin the bloodstream. The waste, which is primarily nitrogen and uric acid mixed in a small amount of water, passes into a pouch in the center of the kidney, where it is collected. The urine then moves down through the ureters, muscular tubes about the diameter of a pencil, that run along the spine. The muscular walls of the ureters actively contract in order to push the urine down and into the bladder.

WHAT DOES THE BLADDER LOOK LIKE?

The bladder is a soft, tan-colored muscle shaped like a hollow ball. When it is empty, it collapses to about the size of an orange. As it fills, the muscle stretches and the walls get thinner. When it is

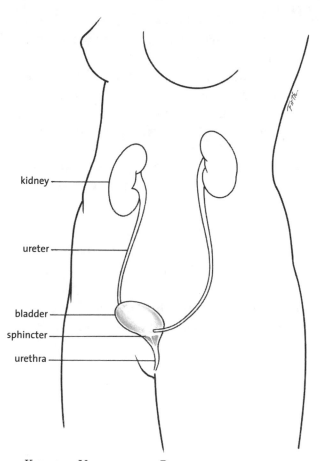

Figure 2-1: KIDNEYS, URETERS, AND BLADDER

completely full, it holds about 20 ounces of urine and is about the size of a large grapefruit.

The bladder lies in the front of your lower abdomen, right behind the pubic bone. The front part of the bladder connects to the urethra, the small (about 1¹/₂ inches long), muscular tube that carries urine outside your body. The muscle that keeps the urine held in the bladder, called the sphincter muscle, can be found where the bladder connects to the urethra. This area, called the bladder neck, contains blood vessels and collagen fibers that work together to keep the bladder closed. If these parts don't work correctly, incontinence may occur.

Muscles and connective tissue, called fascia, connect to the bones on either side of the pelvis, forming a sling that holds the bladder in place. Figure 1-1 illustrates the normal positions of the bladder, uterus, and rectum. Damage to the muscles or fascia, sometimes as a result of childbirth, straining, or aging, can alter the position of the bladder or urethra and can lead to stress incontinence. Chapter 4 details the relationship between childbirth and the health of the bladder.

WHAT DO THE INSIDES OF THE BLADDER AND URETHRA LOOK LIKE?

A cystoscope, a small telescope about half the diameter of a pencil, can be placed inside the urethra and bladder in order to see inside them (Figure 2-2). The lining of the urethra has small, soft, pink

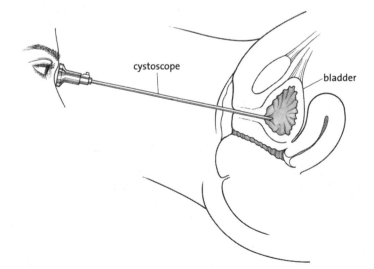

Figure 2-2: CYSTOSCOPY

folds that press against each other to form a pliable seal that helps keep it closed. When the cystoscope is inserted, it gently pushes these folds apart so that your physician can see the urethra and the bladder. At the point where the urethra connects to the bladder (the bladder neck) the urethra narrows as a result of pressure from the surrounding muscles. These muscles, called the urethral sphincter, are normally contracted and work to keep the urethra closed. As the cystoscope is gently guided past this narrowing, it enters the bladder.

Glistening mucous cells lining the inside of the bladder protect the pinkish colored tissues from the mild acidity of the urine. When the bladder empties and collapses, the lining cells form many folds of tissue that look like sand dunes. As the bladder fills, these folds stretch and start to disappear. When the bladder is totally full, its inside looks smooth and round. At the bottom of the bladder, two small dimples can be seen, one on either side. This is where the ureters enter the bladder to empty urine from the kidneys. The ureters are muscular tubes that gently propel the urine down to the bladder in waves of contractions. If you watch closely through the cystoscope, you can actually see the urine spurt out of the openings in the center of each dimple.

As is true with most parts of the body, the colors and shapes inside the bladder and urethra are pleasing and interesting. When using the cystoscope to diagnose problems, we can appreciate the beauty and complexity of the human body.

DO YOU REALLY NEED TO DRINK ALL THAT WATER?

We don't know exactly how everyone got so concerned about drinking lots of water, but many theories have it that extra water keeps your kidneys functioning well, keeps you from overeating, and keeps your skin healthy. Not surprisingly, the International Bottled

Water Association promotes these ideas aggressively. However, your kidneys are designed to work without a flood of water, and there is no medical evidence that more water helps them work any better. Some women think that drinking a lot of water helps curb the appetite, but studies show that drinking lots of extra water does not lead to a decrease in the total number of calories people eat in a day. There are no studies that show that water helps with weight loss. Let's face it, no one's appetite is satisfied by just drinking water. There is also no evidence to show that drinking a lot of water helps keep your skin moist and healthy. Dermatologists suggest that if your skin seems dry, you should apply lotion, not drink extra water.

Your body is well designed to tell you exactly how much fluid you need in a day; this mechanism is called thirst! Your brain very accurately senses when there is not enough water in your system and then tells you to find something to drink. If you are dehydrated from sweating, your thirst tells you to drink what you lost. If you drink when you're thirsty, you'll get the right amount. Around four 8-ounce glasses of fluids a day, all told, is enough. In fact, most people get enough water in the foods they eat during a normal day to satisfy the body's need for fluids. Fruits, vegetables, meat, fish, poultry, and dairy products all contain lots of water.

Ida and Pearl's Problems with Water

Ida and Pearl are sisters and longtime patients in our practice. Pearl, age sixty, came in for a checkup but spoke more about her sister than she did about herself. "My big sister, Ida, is extreme in everything, and when it comes to her health, she's a fanatic. If you tell her that eating spinach once a week is good for your health, she'll eat it ten times a week. Now she's on a water kick. She read somewhere that drinking eight glasses of water a day is good for your health, so she's drinking twelve! I don't even know how she can get it all down. Is drinking all that water bad for her?"

We assured Pearl that while Ida's new water-drinking habit was extreme, it wouldn't injure anything. Nonetheless, drinking excessive amounts of water puts an unnecessary strain on the bladder and might cause Ida to lose control occasionally. Pearl was relieved but vowed to "set Ida straight and make sure she stops this craziness."

Two months later Ida, age sixty-two, came in for her regular checkup. She told us she was feeling fine but shyly added that there was "one small problem." She explained that she was "simply following the instructions in all the magazines about the importance of drinking lots of water but am embarrassed because I wet my pants quite a bit."

We talked about exactly how much water is really needed each day. Ida told us she was drinking "a bit more than that." We suggested she cut back her consumption and let us know if the incontinence resolved.

Three weeks later Ida called with the good news that she is always dry. "My sister Pearlie drives me crazy. But the truth is, she's usually right. My water-drinking marathon is over."

HOW DO YOU NORMALLY
CONTROL YOUR BLADDER?

Your brain has a complicated task when it comes to controlling your bladder. In order for the bladder to work properly, your brain must first allow the bladder to fill with urine without any awareness on your part. Then, when the bladder is reasonably full, holding about 7 ounces, the brain needs to warn you that you will have to urinate soon. When the bladder holds about 10 to 15 ounces of urine, your brain tells you to find a bathroom, fast.

You are used to your brain sending signals to the muscles of your body when you want to use them. When you are not using a muscle, it is generally relaxed. However, the brain's control of the bladder is much more complicated. For starters, the bladder and the urethral sphincter must work in opposition to each other. When the bladder is filling and relaxed, the sphincter must be contracted to hold the urine in. When you wish to empty your bladder, the sphincter must relax while the bladder contracts to push the urine out. There are about a dozen intricate pathways back and forth from the brain to the spinal cord nerves, and from the spinal cord nerves to the bladder and sphincter, that coordinate this activity. And almost all of these signals occur without your conscious thought.

Once you reach the bathroom, you intentionally relax the sphincter in order to urinate. However, this process is not so simple either. Right after you consciously relax the sphincter, a reflex (by definition, something that is not under your control) occurs that causes the bladder muscle to contract in order to push the urine out. Another reflex causes the pelvic muscles supporting the bladder to relax in order to relieve any resistance to the urine coming out. When your bladder is empty, the sphincter closes, the bladder relaxes, and the pelvic muscles contract. Then the process starts all over again. And you thought urinating was simple!

CAN ANY OF THESE AREAS MALFUNCTION?

If any of the nerves going to the bladder or sphincter is damaged, the normal but complicated series of events involved in emptying your bladder may be compromised. If the area of the brain that allows the bladder to relax is damaged, the signals that make it contract overwhelm the bladder, which goes into spasms. If the brain or the nerves that carry the signals to the sphincter are not working properly, the sphincter may stay open and leak urine constantly. On the other end of the spectrum, if the brain's signals to the sphincter ordering relaxation are not working, the bladder may not be able to push the urine out past these muscles. If this happens, you may not be able to empty your bladder.

There are a number of conditions that can affect the areas of the brain that control urination or the nerves that carry signals to the bladder. Brain injury, stroke, diabetes, multiple sclerosis, and Parkinson's disease are among them. An accident resulting in trauma to the pelvis or injury to the bladder nerves (as sometimes occurs with childbirth) can also interfere with normal urination. If your doctor suspects that any of these conditions is responsible for a bladder problem, he or she can perform specialized tests to fully determine the nature of the problem.

HOW ELSE DOES THE BLADDER NORMALLY PREVENT URINE FROM LEAKING OUT?

The bladder and urethra have a number of mechanisms, other than the nerves and muscles, that are responsible for holding urine in until you are ready to release it. One mechanism to keep urine in the bladder involves the small blood vessels surrounding the urethra. These vessels are normally filled with blood, thus compressing the urethral opening and helping it stay closed. In general, estrogen helps to dilate blood vessels and improve blood flow to many organs. Without adequate estrogen, blood flow decreases and the vessels collapse, allowing the urethral opening to enlarge (see Figure 1-3). Then urine can be lost more easily.

A second way in which estrogen improves bladder function is by helping to keep collagen fibers healthy. Collagen fibers surrounding the urethra make up a spongy bed that helps to support the urethra. When the muscle, collagen, and blood vessels work well, they compress the bladder neck and keep it properly closed. Incontinence can occur if any of these parts doesn't function properly.

WHAT DOES THE FUTURE HOLD?

Medicine is changing quickly. The promises of new systems to deliver medication in ways that mimic normal body function, methods to grow organs starting from stem cells, and genetic engineering to avoid the development of disease in the first place are all on the horizon. While we may be years away from these developments, today's medicine has quite a bit to offer. We need to do our best to keep our bodies in good working order. When a problem arises, we need to find the best treatments available. This book is designed to help you do just that.

CHAPTER 3

Diagnosing Incontinence

Susan's Story

"Grammy, my *Tyrannosaurus rex* is going to eat you up!" shouted exuberant six-year-old Will as he came running into the living room. Will had dressed his little black-and-white dog in a green cloth and a pointy green hat left over from a birthday party. Wiggling and wagging, Will and his "T-Rex" burst into the room. Susan delighted in her grandson's antics and started giggling. Getting just the response he'd hoped for, Will kept roaring and charging and posing with his happily confused puppy. Susan felt a cautionary urge and shushed Will, pleading, "I'm laughing so hard I'm going to tinkle." What could be better as far as Will was concerned? He continued his dinosaur attack, trying harder and harder to be fierce and funny. Susan quickly stood up, repeating, "I'm going to tinkle" all the way to the bathroom. By this time, she sounded irritated. Will looked up with a puzzled look on his face. "Grammy, Grammy, wait! My Tyrannosaurus wants to show you something." "Not now!" Susan scolded as she scurried out. In the safety of the bathroom, she felt relief. "Whew, that was close. I'm glad I made it," she thought. But the relief faded fast. "Oh, poor Will. I know I hurt his feelings. Why can't I just enjoy a good laugh with my grandson? Why do I always have to worry about wetting my pants?"

HOW CAN THE DOCTOR TELL WHICH TYPE OF INCONTINENCE YOU HAVE?

Incontinence is usually evaluated by a doctor with a special interest in this problem, generally a gynecologist, urologist, or urogynecologist (see Chapter 13). The first part of figuring out what kind of incontinence you have should be a discussion with your doctor about exactly what causes *you* to lose urine. Expect to be asked a lot of questions. Just put any sense of discomfort or embarrassment aside and answer as completely as you can. Your answers are part of the information the doctor needs to determine the type of problem you have. It is a good idea to think carefully about these things even before you see the doctor. Some doctors may send you a questionnaire before your appointment so that you arrive at the office with all the information at hand. The questions your doctor will ask are probably among the ones we've written below. It might help if you go through these questions and bring the answers with you when you visit your doctor.

What Activities Cause You to Leak?

Loss of urine upon laughing, coughing, or sneezing often indicates stress incontinence. Loss of urine when you change position or when you put your hands in water often indicates urgency incontinence.

Is the Amount of Urine Lost Small, or Do You Flood?

Stress incontinence usually causes leakage of a small amount of urine, while urgency incontinence can cause the loss of a lot of urine.

Do You Wear Panty Liners, Pads, or Adult Diapers to Protect Your Clothes from Wetting?

Your answer tells the doctor the severity of the problem.

Do You Have an Urge to Urinate Before You Lose Any Urine?

A strong urge to go, followed by a loss of urine, is usually a sign of urgency incontinence. With stress incontinence, you do not feel any urge.

Do You Lose Urine Before You Get to the Bathroom?

This is usually associated with an uncontrollable urge to go and indicates urgency incontinence.

Do These Urges Occur Only with a Full Bladder?

If incontinence happens only with a full bladder, perhaps you are drinking too much or not going to the bathroom frequently enough.

How Often Do You Urinate During the Day? During the Night?

Most people urinate about six times during the day and once at night. An overactive bladder may lead to urgency and make you feel that you have to urinate more frequently.

Does Your Bladder Feel Empty After You Urinate?

Scarring of the urethra may prevent you from emptying your bladder. An overactive bladder feels irritated much of the time and may never feel empty.

Is There Pain or Burning When You Urinate?

These are often signs of a bladder infection.

Do You Get More Than One or Two Bladder Infections a Year?

Chronic or recurrent infections can cause long-lasting problems with the bladder.

Do You Have Any Difficulty Starting a Stream of Urine?

This might indicate a blockage in the urethra or a problem with the nerves leading to the bladder.

Do You Have Any Trouble Stopping the Flow of Urine Once It Starts?

Urgency incontinence can cause this symptom.

Do You Feel Any Bulging from the Vagina?

As a result of weakened pelvic tissue, the bladder may bulge down (cystocele) or the rectum may bulge up (rectocele) in the vagina. You may feel pressure in the vagina from this or may even feel the bulging at the opening of the vagina.

Do You Feel a Pulling or Pressure in the Pelvis, Especially When You Are on Your Feet for Any Length of Time?

This symptom may indicate prolapse.

Do You Leak Constantly?

Intrinsic sphincter deficiency (ISD) or overflow incontinence can cause this symptom (see Chapter 1).

Do You Have Any Neurological Problems, Especially of the Lower Back or Legs?

A severe injury to your back, a stroke, Parkinson's disease, or multiple sclerosis may interfere with the function of your bladder.

Do You Have Diabetes?

Diabetes can cause damage to the nerves going to the bladder, which may cause the bladder not to work as well as it should.

Have You Previously Had Bladder Surgery?

Surgery may have caused scar tissue that can interfere with the proper closure of the urethra.

Your answers to these questions will help give your doctor an idea as to what type of incontinence you might have. Think carefully about the questions, and take the answers to your doctor. The next step in fixing the problem is a physical examination.

Marcy's Story

Marcy is a retired business executive who fell in love with farming and travel. At the age of seventy, she moved to a remote coastal town in a rural area of Spain. "I've got olive trees, vegetables, and a small herd of goats, plus all of Spain to explore. I'm in heaven." Since her family remained in California, she hires a caretaker for her farm and comes to the United States annually for an extended vacation. She also uses the visit to have medical and dental checkups done. Four years ago, Marcy complained to another gynecologist about leaking during physical activity. He noticed some prolapse during the evaluation and decided that surgery would help. Unfortunately, after the surgery Marcy had a new kind of leakage. She did not leak with activity any longer, but now she got a strong urge to urinate and then dribbled on the way to the bathroom. After urinating, she did not feel empty and would soon get another urge to go and would leak again on the way back to the toilet. In order to empty at all, she had to position herself and maneuver in different directions. She described it as her "toilet dance."

A complete exam and evaluation revealed that while Marcy's previous surgery had cured her stress incontinence, it had suspended her bladder too high, and she could not empty it. The too-high suspension resulted in bladder spasms and urge incontinence. We recommended surgical removal of the stitches from the last operation, a procedure that would allow the bladder to return to its normal position. Then we would place a sling under the bladder to support it.

Marcy understood the mechanics of the plan and

thought it sounded good. With what she called "faith in the best medical care in the world," Marcy underwent the procedures we recommended. After a six-week recuperation period at her daughter's house, Marcy was ready for the farm and her goats. She returned to Spain, her "toilet dance" nothing but a memory.

WHAT CAN YOUR DOCTOR TELL FROM AN EXAMINATION?

Your doctor will perform the first examination for incontinence or prolapse in the same way as all gynecologic exams are done. The doctor will have you lie on your back on the examining table with your feet in stirrups. The uterus, fallopian tubes, and ovaries will be examined to make sure they feel normal. Even if you have had a hysterectomy, the doctor will perform an internal exam to make sure nothing else is pushing down on the vagina or rectum. The vagina will then be examined a bit more carefully to see if the bladder or rectum is pushing against a weakened vaginal wall, causing a visible bulge. You will be asked to cough or bear down so that any weakness in the muscles supporting the bladder or rectum is made more apparent. The extra pressure will make weakened areas bulge further. Childbirth, gravity, menopause, aging, and heredity may all contribute to the problem of sagging or dropping of these organs.

The areas around the vagina and rectum will be touched with a Q-tip, and the doctor will record your ability to feel that touch. If you are unable to feel the Q-tip touching you, there may be a problem with the nerves in the area of the bladder or rectum. In that case, you may be referred to a neurologist for further evaluation. Some neurological conditions, such as back injuries, strokes, diabetes, and multiple sclerosis, can affect the muscles that aid bladder function.

You will need to stand up for the next part of the exam. Although this may sound odd, a dropped bladder or uterus may be apparent only when you are standing. This standing exam is completely painless. With one of your feet elevated on a stool, the doctor can observe any bulging from the dropping of the uterus, bladder, or rectum. There is a new way to record this information, called POPQ (pronounced "pop-Q"), which stands for *p*elvic *o*rgan *p*rolapse— *q*uantitative. This system standardizes the measurements so that every doctor measures things the same way. Since the POPQ is new and detailed, many doctors have yet to start using it.

WHAT ARE THE Q-TIP TEST, STRESS TEST, AND ULTRASOUND EVALUATION?

After the pelvic examination, other tests may be employed to help determine which type of incontinence you have. We routinely perform two simple tests called the cough stress test and the Q-tip test. The cough stress test is performed with you lying on the exam table with your feet in stirrups. You are asked to cough with a full bladder to see if that causes leakage of urine. The Q-tip test is performed in the same position. A cotton-tipped swab covered with anesthetic gel is painlessly inserted into the urethra, the bladder opening. You are asked to cough and strain, and the doctor or nurse measures the movement of the end of the Q-tip (Figure 3-1). Excessive movement of the Q-tip or loss of urine with coughing usually indicates a weakening of the tissues supporting the urethra that is associated with *stress* incontinence.

Next, you will be asked to empty your bladder completely. A small tube, called a *catheter,* is painlessly passed through the urethra into the bladder, and any remaining urine is collected and measured. The amount of urine left in the bladder after urination is called the postvoid residual. Some doctors now use ultrasound to measure the postvoid residual and the amount of movement of the

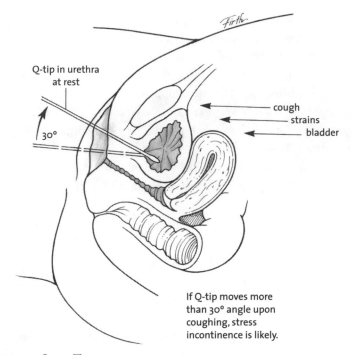

Q-tip in urethra
at rest

30°

Firth

cough
strains
bladder

If Q-tip moves more
than 30° angle upon
coughing, stress
incontinence is likely.

Figure 3-1: Q-TIP TEST

urethra upon a laugh or a cough. The only part of the instrument that touches you is a small wand placed in the vagina, just beneath the bladder.

Almost everyone has some urine remaining in the bladder after a trip to the bathroom, even if you feel you have entirely emptied it. It is normal to have up to two ounces left over. More indicates that your bladder is not able to empty properly. This is often associated with a type of incontinence called *overflow incontinence.* Overflow incontinence can be the result of problems with the nerves that signal the bladder or scar tissue blocking the flow of urine out of the bladder (see Chapter 1). A sample of urine from the catheter is usually sent to the laboratory and cultured to test for infection. If there is an infection, it is treated with antibiotics.

WHAT IS A VOIDING DIARY?

During the first office visit, your doctor will probably ask you how often you urinate, how much liquid you drink in a day, and how often you have accidents. The answers to these questions are a good start, but a written record of these events may more specifically illustrate what happens with your bladder during the course of your day. This written record is called a *voiding diary*, or urolog. It is intended to be a one- or two-day record of how much liquid you drink, the amount and frequency of your urination, and how much leaking you have. Because a written record is better than relying on your memory, the voiding diary is a very accurate method of determining just how significant the incontinence problem is. All of the patients in our practice fill out a voiding diary (Figure 3-2).

In the left-hand column is a place to record the date and time when you have anything to drink. The amount and kind of liquid are recorded in the next column. The third column is the place to record the times you urinate during the day and night and the amount of urine passed. The amount of urine is often measured with a special basin that fits under the seat of any toilet. The basin has ounces marked on it, and you simply read off the amount and record it in your voiding diary. The urine is then discarded in the toilet and flushed away. The voiding diary also has a column for you to record any accidents you have during the two days. Your doctor needs to know if you have an urge to void before you leak or if the leaking occurs without any warning.

The voiding diary is important because it gives the doctor an idea of what your problem is like in real life. It can also point out medical problems, and sometimes it helps us find a "lifestyle" rather than a medical or surgical solution. After treatment, we may ask you to keep the diary again to see exactly how the solution works for you.

Directions: Please complete the information listed below for two (2) consecutive twenty-four-hour periods.

- Begin with first urination upon arising.
- Record intake amount in ounces and type of fluid (i.e., coffee, tea, juice, water, etc.)
- Record urine output and time of void. Measure in container provided.
- Record intake/output for two (2) days. Remember to record both day and night.

| | INTAKE RECORD | | OUTPUT RECORD | | |
Date	Time of Intake (A.M./P.M.)	Amount of Fluid Intake (oz.)	Time of Void (A.M./P.M.)	Amount Voided (oz.)	Accidents

Figure 3-2: VOIDING DIARY

Judy's Story

Judy is a forty-six-year-old mother of two young girls. Before starting her family, Judy worked in children's theater workshops. She composed songs, wrote dialogue, and arranged and produced stage shows for schools and community centers. Now that Judy is perpetually busy with her children, the only time peaceful and quiet enough to even think about her music is at night after the dishes are washed, the lunches for the next day made, and the kids asleep in their beds. "I live for those late nights in a quiet house with just my music and no interruptions," Judy almost whispered. But lately she had been waking up on cold, wet sheets. Initially she talked herself into believing that she must be having hot flashes in her sleep, which soaked the sheets with sweat. "Gee, I guess this is menopause," she remarked one morning. But her husband, Paul, thought it might be something else: "I hate to say this, honey, but I think you wet the bed." That day she called us for an appointment.

As the first step in her medical evaluation, we asked Judy to keep a voiding diary, which painted a clearer picture of her problem. The excitement of composing and writing again inspired Judy to stay up late three or four nights a week. The mugs of steaming coffee she drank helped too! At around nine at night, Judy would start drinking strong black coffee. By the time she fell into bed at around 1 A.M., she'd consumed about three full mugs. Despite all that caffeine, she usually dropped off into a deep sleep. When Paul got up at 6 A.M., Judy would find herself on her cold, damp side of the bed. We decided that a bladder spasm emptied her very full bladder sometime shortly before she woke up. The coffee was the source of her very full bladder, and the caffeine was a likely bladder irritant. As she was exhausted from staying up so late, the call of her irritated and full bladder wasn't waking her soon enough. Judy was able to see this pattern, and we were able to figure out a solution. Judy didn't want to give up her "private time," so we suggested she cut down on the coffee, switch to half decaf, half caffeinated, and set an alarm for 5 A.M. to make a quick trip to the bathroom before her bladder became overfull.

Judy played with the solution until she found the right mix. The coffee was vital to keeping her awake and working at night, but two cups, not three (only one with 100 percent caffeine), was enough. As much as she hated to set a 5 A.M. alarm, she was able to fall back asleep right after her trip to the bathroom and generally stayed asleep, dry and warm, until the girls called her at around 7 A.M.

WHAT IS A PAD COUNT?

Some women wear pads to protect their underwear and clothes from urine leakage. Your doctor will probably ask you about this during the office visit. The size and absorbency of pads vary, as does the frequency that women change them during the day. In order to accurately measure the amount of urine you may be losing during the day, some doctors ask you to do a pad count. For a day or two before your appointment, you will be asked to keep all the pads you use in a sealed plastic bag and bring them, along with one dry pad, to the doctor's office. This is not the most pleasant task, but it does tell the doctor exactly how much urine you are losing during the day. We weigh the wet pads, then the single dry one, and calculate how much urine you have lost. In addition to measuring the number of pads you use during a day, the test can also calculate if whatever treatment we prescribe actually decreases the amount of urine lost.

WHAT IS URODYNAMICS TESTING?

In order for us to understand what is causing your incontinence, we sometimes need to figure out if the bladder muscle is working properly. The test for this is known as *urodynamics,* or UDS for short. Despite the peculiar name, this has nothing to do with jet planes or aerodynamics. The term urodynamics implies that we are able to see the bladder (uro), in action (dynamic). The muscular sac we call the bladder is supposed to stay relaxed and then comfortably expand while it collects and stores urine made by the kidneys. The bladder is supposed to work without any effort, or even awareness, on your part. Then, when you are ready to urinate, it should contract and force the urine out. The urodynamic study allows us to measure the way the bladder works: Does it fill up without the contractions associated with overactivity? Does it contract properly and at the right time? Can the bladder hold a reasonable amount of urine? Does it hold too little urine? Too much? When it contracts, does it get all the urine out?

UDS testing allows us to answer these questions. Some women may need to have UDS testing done, especially if the diagnosis is not clear to the doctor after the initial tests described above. UDS testing is performed in the office, takes about one hour, and is painless. Your doctor will ask you to undress from the waist down and wrap a sheet around your waist. First you will sit in a special chair that supports your back, buttocks, and legs in a comfortable position. This chair allows your doctor to tilt you back to a lying position in order to perform the first part of the testing. Then, without your having to move, you can be tilted to a sitting position to see if your bladder functions any differently while you are upright—as you are for most of the day. The first part of the testing involves urinating into a specialized basin that measures how fast or slowly the urine comes out of your bladder. If something is blocking the urine, such as scarring inside the urethra or a bladder muscle that isn't working properly, the flow will be slow. If the urethra is held wide open by scar tissue, as sometimes happens following a previous bladder operation, the flow will be faster than normal because the urethra cannot hold the urine in. This part of UDS testing is called the *urine flow test*.

After the urine flow test, your doctor will measure the way your bladder works as it fills, how it works when you laugh, cough, or sneeze, and how it works when you try to empty it. The following description of this part of the test sounds like "weird science," but our patients assure us that while it is a bit strange and sounds complicated, it is not at all uncomfortable. Before the procedure, a nurse painlessly places a very small tube in the bladder, another very small tube in the rectum, and a small, spongy specialized tampon in the vagina. Each of the tubes and the tampon are attached by wires to a computer that measures the functioning of the three areas (Figure 3-3).

The first part of the test measures how much urine is left in the bladder after you urinate. This is called the postvoid residual. Your doctor will then use the tube in the bladder to slowly fill it with ster-

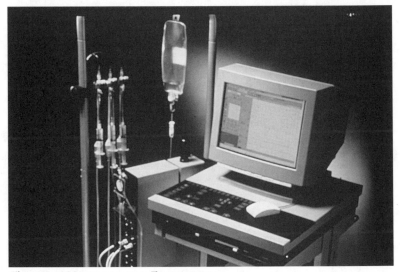

Figure 3-3: URODYNAMICS EQUIPMENT

ile water. You should not be able to feel anything until your bladder gets filled to the point where you would normally have to urinate. Your doctor will ask you to tell us when this is. Then your doctor will ask you to cough (or bear down) after the addition of every 3 ounces of fluid from that point forward, to see if you leak. Leaking is a sign of having stress incontinence. Your doctor will continue to fill your bladder and ask you to say when you are really full—the point when, if you were driving, you might pull off the road to find a bathroom. Shortly thereafter you will feel that you cannot hold any more, and the test will be stopped. The computer measures how much fluid has been put into the bladder and what the pressure is in the bladder as it fills up.

Normally, the bladder expands quietly as it fills, without any contractions at all, until you are ready to empty it. For some women, however, an overactive bladder contracts during the time it is filling. These contractions can be seen on the computer and are recorded for later analysis. An overactive bladder is usually treated nonsurgically. You can read more about treatment for overactive bladders in Chapter 5.

The next part of the test is a repeat of the first part, but in a sitting position. Because most women with incontinence lose urine in the standing or sitting position, this part of the test may reveal problems that were not apparent when you were lying down. During this part of the UDS, a test called the *abdominal leak point pressure test* is also performed. After your bladder is partly filled, you will be asked to bear down as hard as you can. The pressure generated by your abdominal muscles when you bear down pushes on the bladder and increases the pressure inside the bladder. Your doctor will look to see if you lose urine and then measure the pressure in the bladder when this happens. If the mechanisms that normally keep you from leaking are all working, you should not leak despite the increase in pressure. If you leak just as you start to bear down, it is called a *low leak point pressure*. A low leak point pressure usually means that scar tissue is holding the urethra open. Treatment for this problem, called intrinsic sphincter deficiency (ISD), is discussed in Chapter 6.

At this point the testing will be over, and the information your doctor needs to help you should be available. Your doctor will probably ask you to come back a week later to discuss the findings. This allows him or her time to analyze the test results, pull them together with what was found during the physical exam, and create a plan for treatment.

Sandra's Story

"He's getting heavy as a horse, but this is ridiculous." Sandra is a thirty-two-year-old Mexico City native with an active two-year-old boy named César. Sandra spends her days chasing and lifting César as he runs from activity to activity, on the brink of one near disaster after another. "Did I tell you about the time he nearly fell off the boardwalk at the beach?" she asked. "I had to make a mad dash and scoop him up before he took a horrible fall from six feet up." To add to her worries, each time she lifted César, she lost a bit of urine. At first she assumed that the problem would go away. Since he turned two and is now much bigger and faster, the problem had worsened. Sandra had to wear pads every day and found herself dribbling urine upon the lightest activity—rising from a chair, bending to pick up a toy, making a grab for César. "I feel old before my time. Even my mother doesn't have this problem the way I do," she complained. "I'd also like to have my tubes tied. Two children are enough. Sometimes too much."

When we performed Sandra's pelvic exam, we noticed that she had some dropping of the bladder, called a cystocele. We also noticed that her bladder bulged even further in her vagina when she strained or coughed. We did urodynamic studies on Sandra that week. The studies showed that her bladder sphincter (muscle) did not stay closed properly, confirming the diagnosis of stress incontinence. We suggested an outpatient surgery using tension-free vaginal tape (TVT) that would help support her urethra to fix the dropped bladder. She also asked us to tie her tubes at the same time.

Sandra's mother came from Mexico City to help with the children for a couple of weeks. Grandma was happy to see her grandchildren, and Sandra was very happy to say good-bye to the bulky pads. Her surgery was done with TVT, a nylon-like tape that is put under the urethra for support to correct the dropped bladder (see Chapter 6). The surgery, followed by two weeks of recovery, made Sandra's stress incontinence a thing of the past, and now she happily chases César without the pads and without the worry.

IS URODYNAMICS (UDS) TESTING NECESSARY?

Many doctors feel they are able to tell the kind of bladder problem you are having based upon your answers to the questions and the examination in the office. However, a recent study found this approach to diagnosis much less than 100 percent accurate. The researchers asked a bladder specialist to look at the records of more than three hundred women who had bladder problems, with the exception of the results of urodynamic tests that were also performed. The specialist diagnosed one hundred women with stress incontinence based on answers to the doctor's questions and physical examination. But a careful look at the urodynamics testing showed that only thirty-eight of those women really had pure stress incontinence. The other women had either an overactive bladder or a mixture of stress incontinence and an overactive bladder.

Of the eighty-five women thought to have only an overactive bladder, based on the answers to the questions and the exam, only eighteen actually did. The other women had stress incontinence or a combination of the two problems when the UDS testing was evaluated. And of the fifty-six women thought to have mixed incontinence, only eleven had this diagnosis confirmed by urodynamics testing. The other women had either an overactive bladder or pure stress incontinence. Therefore, examination and history alone are often not enough to make the correct diagnosis of bladder problems. Because a correct diagnosis is crucial to planning the proper treatment, urodynamics testing is necessary for most women with incontinence.

WHAT IS VIDEO URODYNAMICS TESTING?

Urodynamics testing tells us about the pressures inside the bladder and urethra, but it does not tell us what the bladder and urethra look like when the bladder is filling or emptying. Some research centers have been testing video urodynamics equipment, which allows the physician to see the bladder on X ray as it fills, holds fluid and empties. By comparing this X-ray picture with the actual pressures recorded at the same time by the urodynamics instruments, they can get a good picture of how the bladder is actually working.

If the flow of urine out of the urethra is blocked, the video reveals where the blockage is. If the bladder and urethra are not working properly to let the urine out, the video may show the urethra closing when it is supposed to open. If the urethra is not strong enough to hold the urine in the bladder, the video shows it spread open, with urine leaking out. The video urodynamics equipment is very expensive, and for most women the additional information it makes available does not help to diagnose the problem. Therefore, your doctor may choose not to perform this test.

WHAT IS CYSTOSCOPY?

Some doctors also perform a cystoscopy as part of the evaluation of incontinence. A cystoscope is a small telescope that can be easily inserted through the urethra and into the bladder. Fluid runs through the telescope and keeps the bladder open and clear, so the doctor can see the lining of the bladder and the opening of the ureters into the bladder. Growths on the lining, such as benign polyps or cancerous tumors, can be seen and biopsied. Sutures incorrectly placed inside the bladder during previous surgery, which often lead to bladder irritation and urgency incontinence, can be seen with the cystoscope. Other conditions, such as interstitial cystitis (see Chapter 7) or chronic infection, may be diagnosed. The openings of the ureters can be inspected to see if urine is moving freely into the bladder, confirming that the kidneys and ureters are working properly.

WHAT IS AN IVP?

In some situations, it is important to get an idea of what the bladder, kidneys, and ureters (the tubes that bring the urine from the kidneys to the bladder) look like. While video urodynamics testing shows the bladder and the urethra well, that test does not show the kidneys or ureters at all. One way to get a look is with a procedure called an IVP. A special solution is injected into a vein in your arm and then an X ray is taken of your kidneys, ureters, and bladder. The injected solution collects in the urine as it forms in the kidneys and shows up on the X ray as the urine flows from the kidneys, down the ureters, and into the bladder. The X ray shows the shape and size of these organs and allows the doctor to see any abnormalities that may be present. Blockage of the ureters or urethra, or leakage of urine from the bladder, may be identified.

Fortunately, today your doctors have a number of tools to help figure out the underlying problem. All insurance companies, Medicare, and HMOs cover these tests. Some women may require a few of these tests; others may require many. Your doctor should discuss with you which tests will be necessary to make the diagnosis. Usually, after two or three visits to the doctor's office, the tests can be completed, a diagnosis established, and treatment options discussed with you.

CHAPTER 4

Childbirth and Incontinence

Phoebe's Story

"I'm willing to do whatever it takes to fix this," said Phoebe when she came into our office about four years ago. This beautiful, thirty-four-year-old redhead was at the end of her rope due to incontinence. "It is strangling my life," she said. She had immigrated from England ten years before, married a local man who worked as a hairdresser, and was now the mother of two young children. Her first child weighed 8½ pounds at birth, and Phoebe had a long and tiring labor. She had pushed for two and a half hours before delivering a healthy baby girl they named Cara. Following delivery, Phoebe had some mild urinary loss when she laughed or coughed, but the problem went away almost completely after about six months' time with the help of Kegel exercises. She was able to maintain control over her bladder most of the time, and life went back to normal.

Phoebe's second pregnancy went smoothly, and the labor was a bit easier than with her first child. The delivery was hard, though, and the doctor needed to use forceps to deliver her nine-pound son, Gerald. Phoebe again experienced urinary loss after Gerald's birth but assumed it would go away as it had done with her first child. When we saw her, Gerald was two years old, and Phoebe's urinary loss had gotten worse. She had already given up aerobics classes, and she leaked with nearly every cough, sneeze, or laugh.

Phoebe was a waitress in a pub that catered to British expatriates, and she was seriously thinking about quitting her job. She was on her feet from midday until late evening and needed to change a large pad every few hours to get through the day. Since many of the customers knew her well, she often took a lot of ribbing over her red hair and having married a Yank. The atmosphere was friendly, boisterous, and often funny.

In fact, the incident that sent her in search of help started with a big laugh. One evening, as she was bringing a tray of drinks to a table, she overheard Ian, a frequent customer who was a hangdog, broke, out-of-work store clerk, tell a pretty newcomer that he was a pilot for British Airways flying out to the Bahamas the next day. Phoebe made it past Ian and burst out laughing when she got back to the bar. But the laugh was costly; her (fortunately) dark-colored pants were now good and wet, and her shift was not over for an hour. Phoebe called our office the next day.

When we took her medical history, the difficult labor with her first child and difficult delivery with the second stood out as warning signs of possible damage to her urinary system. Our examination showed that there was a weakness of the pelvic muscles supporting her bladder. We felt that urodynamic testing was needed to be sure there were no other bladder problems. The examination and urodynamics showed that the problem was primarily weakness of her pelvic muscles and ligaments, which allowed the bladder to move out of position when Phoebe laughed, coughed, sneezed, or exerted herself by lifting heavy trays at the pub.

Called *stress incontinence,* this is the most common type of incontinence following childbirth. Phoebe asked what had caused her problem. We answered that although there are a number of things that can lead to damage to the pelvic muscles and nerves, the most common is childbirth. Fortunately, Phoebe could choose from a number of effective treatments.

DOES CHILDBIRTH CAUSE INCONTINENCE?

Everyone who has had a child knows that once that baby is born, life is never the same again. Women also know that their bodies are never exactly the way they were before they gave birth. Recent evidence tells us more precisely how they change. Women who have not delivered a child vaginally rarely develop incontinence or pelvic muscle relaxation, while women who have vaginal deliveries sometimes do. Again, be assured that most women will not go on to develop incontinence after childbirth.

This chapter is to help you understand what we know about why some women who have delivered babies have problems with incontinence. It may also give pause to women yet to deliver or even to conceive. Will their ability to stay dry when they get older be compromised by childbirth? What can they do to prevent it? Understand that we are still at an early stage of fact finding, but we'll nevertheless explore answers to these questions on the pages that follow.

There are many factors that can lead to incontinence: the strength of the pelvic supporting structures you were born with; the forces these structures have resisted over the years, including childbirth, heavy lifting, and straining during bowel movements; your ability to heal if these tissues are injured; the effect of the aging process on the collagen that gives strength to these structures. Probably no one factor is completely responsible for the development of incontinence. Further research is needed to help clarify the importance of each possible cause and the interplay among them, research that will likely benefit women who are yet to have children.

The connection between incontinence and childbirth has been assumed for a long time. When gynecologists see women for problems of incontinence, they are not surprised to find severe problems in women who have had many children or who have delivered large babies. Doctors have started working out the details of these relationships and are looking for the specific reasons why some women go on to develop incontinence and other women never have this problem. Although the studies are preliminary and involve only small numbers of women, details are starting to emerge.

About 10 to 20 percent of women who have a vaginal delivery will be bothered by prolapse—bulging of the bladder, rectum, or uterus into the vagina—by the time they reach the age of fifty. Women who deliver one child have a three times' greater risk of developing prolapse than women who have not had children. Women who delivered two children have a five times' increased risk, and women with four or more children have an eleven times' greater likelihood of developing this problem. Women who need to push longer than one hour to deliver, or who deliver larger babies, appear to be at a greater risk of developing incontinence later in life. There is increasing evidence that childbirth is responsible for much of the injury to the muscles and nerves of the pelvis. This injury eventually leads to urinary loss and pelvic prolapse. Most women are not aware of this somewhat new information. In fact, many doctors are not apprised of the recently collected data. This chapter explains what we know, so far, about incontinence and childbirth.

IS INCONTINENCE COMMON
DURING PREGNANCY?

As the baby grows, the enlarging uterus puts pressure on the bladder below it. This extra stress on the bladder makes it easier for any additional exertion, such as laughing, sneezing, or exercising, to push urine out of the bladder. This is why women often have mild urinary incontinence during pregnancy. During a first pregnancy, more than one third of women develop temporary stress incontinence. During subsequent pregnancies, more than three quarters develop this problem. However, most of the women who have incontinence during pregnancy return to full continence after delivery as the tissues of the birth canal heal. Only about 5 percent of these women still have stress incontinence a year after delivery.

DOES A LONG LABOR LEAD TO INCONTINENCE?

The modern movement of childbirth education is enormously important in helping to educate women about labor, childbirth, breast-feeding and caring for newborns. Doctors rarely have time to talk with their patients in any detail about the steps of labor and childbirth, and childbirth educators fill this need well. Many childbirth educators also focus on avoiding medical interventions that interfere with a "natural" birth, especially cesarean section. Lamaze classes, the Bradley method, and many midwives and doctors encourage women to labor as long as needed and as long as the baby's health, as monitored by the heartbeat, can tolerate labor. As a result, prolonged labor or prolonged pushing is sometimes encouraged in order to avoid a cesarean section. While safe for the baby, it appears these practices may not be in the best long-term interest of the mother. We know now that prolonged and difficult labor may lead to permanent nerve damage and weakening of the pelvic muscles and the supporting structures of the uterus, bladder, and rectum. This can eventually lead to dropping of the pelvic organs or incontinence.

As every woman who delivers a child knows, labor and delivery subject the body to forces that are not encountered in any other circumstance. The muscles and nerves in the pelvis are especially affected. As the baby's head comes down into the pelvis, it presses against the muscles that line the inside of the pelvis. The farther down the baby's head goes into the pelvis, the greater is the pressure against these muscles and underlying nerves. After the cervix is totally dilated, the pushing phase of labor begins. The mother is usually asked to wait for a contraction to start, then hold her breath and bear down as hard as she can in order to push the baby out. This bearing down presses the baby's head against the mother's muscles and nerves to such an extent that the normal flow of blood is cut off temporarily, until that push is over. Without a fresh supply of blood, the tissues are deprived of oxygen and nutrition, making them more susceptible to damage. The pressures generated by pushing are three times as high as the tissues would normally tolerate for any prolonged time. However, the few minutes of rest in between contractions usually lets blood flow back to the area. This fresh blood carries oxygen and nutrition to the muscles and nerves and carries carbon dioxide and waste materials away. The several minutes between contractions are normally enough for the tissue to recover.

However, unless delivery occurs quickly, the baby's head continues to press against the tissues with each contraction. For some women this pressure can cumulatively add up to many hours. Two nerves, called the *pudendal* and the *pelvic* nerves, lie on each side of the birth canal within the muscles that are directly under the baby's head. Because they are so close to the baby's head, these nerves are especially vulnerable to the pressures of labor. The pudendal and pelvic nerves carry the signals from the brain to the muscles that hold the bladder and rectum in place. If these nerves are injured, the signals meant for the muscles around the bladder, vagina, and rectum may not be transmitted properly. Without stimulation from the nerves, the pelvic muscles, like any under-used muscles, can become weak and flaccid. Some studies show changes in the function of these nerves in more than half of women following vaginal delivery. Interestingly, a prolonged labor or pushing phase before a cesarean is performed makes it likely that nerve damage has already occurred—*even if the baby is eventually delivered by cesarean.* Over time and with age, the supporting tissues of the bladder, rectum, and uterus weaken, adding to the injuries associated with childbirth. The result can be incontinence of urine or stool, or prolapse.

Some recent studies show that the likelihood of incontinence and prolapse is lower if the mother (and her doctor) allows the natural force of the uterine contractions to push the baby down the birth canal, rather than the mother pushing as hard as she can during this time. Studies show that if the voluntary pushing part of labor can be limited to less than an hour, there is a lower incidence of injury to the nerves and muscles of the pelvis. This alternative may be a safer and more natural way to deliver. Let the uterus do the work it was designed to do.

CAN VAGINAL DELIVERY LEAD TO INCONTINENCE?

The extraordinary forces on a woman's body during delivery of the baby may damage pelvic tissues. As the baby's head comes out, the forces can actually tear the ligaments that anchor the pelvic supporting muscles to the pelvic bones. The muscles themselves may also be damaged (Figure 4-1). Sometimes the muscle near the outside of the vagina is intentionally cut by the doctor to help speed up the delivery. We now know that this cut, called an episiotomy, increases the risk of anal incontinence.

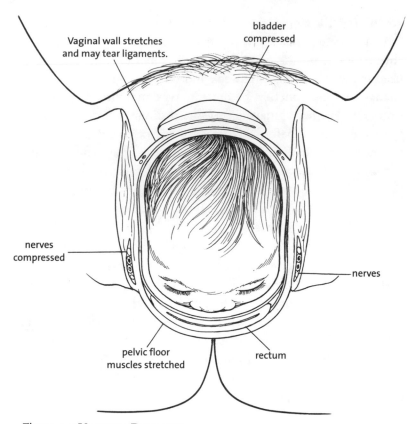

Figure 4-1: VAGINAL DELIVERY

In some women these damaged muscles and ligaments remain weak and do not heal entirely. As time goes on and the normal changes of aging and weakening of the tissues takes place, incontinence may result. At present, only sophisticated and expensive tests such as MRI or nerve conduction studies can tell if these muscles and nerves have returned to normal. Unfortunately, there is no convenient, easy way for you or your doctor to know if these muscles are weakened and destined to lead to incontinence. Nor is there presently any remedy for nerve damage.

WHAT ROLE DOES FORCEPS DELIVERY
PLAY IN INCONTINENCE?

The use of forceps increases the risk of injury to the nerves and muscles of the pelvis. Forceps are the spoon-shaped metal instruments that are sometimes inserted into the mother's vagina and placed around the baby's head at the time of delivery. These instruments are usually used after a long or difficult labor to help deliver a baby. As the doctor pulls on the forceps, they push aside the muscles and soft tissues in the pelvis, allowing more room for the baby to come out. The forceps also help the doctor to pull the baby out, especially if there is a tight fit. However, because the instruments are made of metal and take up space of their own, they increase the risk of stretching and tearing the vagina and supporting tissues of the pelvis. They also increase pressure on the nerves that run inside the pelvis. As a result, more harm can be done to the tissues, possibly resulting in long-term damage and eventual incontinence.

Forceps were invented in the 1500s, at a time when cesarean section was commonly fatal for the mother. Forceps offered women a lifesaving alternative in the event of a difficult birth. The development of forceps is both an innovation and a stain on the history of obstetrics. Forceps were invented by Pierre Chamberlain, a French physician living in England, in the sixteenth century. Despite the urgent need for them, these instruments were kept secret by him and his family for the next three generations, about a hundred years. This secret allowed the Chamberlain family to promote the idea that they were more skilled than other obstetricians and could deliver babies where others had failed. Since medical practitioners outside the Chamberlain family had no knowledge of this lifesaving instrument, many women died needlessly. In the late 1600s, one of the Chamberlains sold the idea of the forceps to another physician, who went on to license their use for a fee.

In time the knowledge of forceps spread, and many obstetricians became trained in their use. The proper use of forceps became a hallmark of trained obstetricians. Midwives were forbidden to use them, and this is still true today. Even in the early 1900s, the risks associated with cesarean section, including infection, bleeding, anesthesia, and death, far outweighed the risks associated with the use of forceps. A forceps delivery was state-of-the-art obstetrics for a time, and many women and children survived childbirth because of them. However, by the late 1900s, surgical and anesthetic techniques improved, antibiotics made infection less dangerous, and blood transfusions prevented many deaths from hemorrhage. These factors made cesarean section safer. In addition, it became apparent that the metal arms of the forceps are not always kind to the baby's head. On rare occasions, small skull fractures can result and sometimes lead to permanent injury to the baby. Consequently, cesarean section became the accepted tool for the obstetrician to use in a long or difficult labor.

Because there is a risk of complications with forceps, they should probably not be used to deliver a baby unless there is a rapid drop in the baby's heartbeat, severe bleeding, or another emergency that dictates a quick delivery. While forceps are used less often now, the use of an instrument called the vacuum extractor has increased in the past ten years. The vacuum extractor may be safer for the mother, but it may not be entirely safe for the baby. This instrument has a soft plastic suction cup that is attached to a handle. The obstetrician applies a suction cup to the top of the baby's head, and it hardly touches the mother at all. The doctor pulls on the handle while the mother pushes, and the combined effort can help deliver the baby. However, recent studies show a very slight increase in the risk of injury to the baby's head with this device. As a result, even the vacuum extractor may be used less in the future.

DO DOCTORS HAVE NONMEDICAL REASONS
TO AVOID CESAREAN SECTIONS?

Up to the recent past, there were incentives for doctors to perform cesarean sections. The fee charged to perform a cesarean was higher than that charged for a vaginal birth. This compensated the physician for the lost time and lost sleep for attending a long, difficult labor. A cesarean section is sometimes a way out of such a labor for the baby, the mother, and the doctor. Most insurance companies used to pay an additional thousand dollars or so for performing a cesarean and caring for the mother in the hospital for a five-day stay while she recovered from surgery. With managed care and the changes in health care, incentives changed. Many insurance companies now pay doctors the same fee whether a cesarean is performed or not. Therefore, the additional time to care for the patient in the hospital for five days and the postoperative office visits have become extra, uncompensated work for the doctor.

Doctors also have other incentives to avoid cesarean sections. Hospitals and managed care groups encourage doctors to keep cesarean section rates low. A cesarean section is expensive for the insurance company. Since it is a surgical procedure, it requires more equipment and resources than a vaginal delivery. Women stay in the hospital longer and need more nursing care, more blood tests, more medication, more supplies, more of everything. The rate of cesareans is easy to calculate: the number of cesareans divided by the number of total deliveries for each doctor. Reducing cesareans is consequently an easy target for managed care bureaucrats. They scrutinize every doctor closely and may have the doctor appear in front of a review committee or even cancel the doctor's contract if the number of cesareans wanders upward over the year. During their formal training, obstetrical residents are taught to keep the cesarean section rate low, both their personal rate and the rate for their group of residents. They are instructed that high numbers of cesarean sections imply poor obstetrical practice, and they are urged to remember the cost-saving realities they will face in the managed care world after completing their obstetrical training. These are the subtle—and not so subtle—pressures that residents and doctors are made to feel in order to keep cesarean section rates low.

Yet recent evidence suggests that some women will end up with urinary or anal incontinence caused by prolonged labor that could be avoided by a cesarean section. It is becoming clear that more, not fewer, cesarean sections might be indicated to help women avoid damage to the pelvic muscles and nerves that help control bladder and rectal function. Cesarean sections might also prevent the need for a number of these women to have surgery in the future to repair the damage done by well-intended, but ill-advised, obstetrical practices. As more information accumulates about childbirth's relationship to incontinence, obstetrical practice may very well change in order to prevent future problems for mothers.

DOES CHILDBIRTH INEVITABLY
LEAD TO INCONTINENCE?

Despite all the forces the pelvic tissues endure during labor and childbirth, incontinence is not inevitable. In fact, a woman's body is remarkably resilient, and the vast majority of women who give birth do not develop incontinence. In most cases, the damage created by childbirth repairs itself over time as the tissues go through the normal healing process. Almost half of all women who have a vaginal delivery show immediate recovery of the nerves' ability to carry messages to the pelvic muscles, and 60 percent have complete resolution within two months. However, in some women the injured tissue does not recover 100 percent of its prelabor strength. For them, the likelihood of incontinence and the possibility of pelvic prolapse developing later in life are more common.

The actual specific risks of developing incontinence vary for individual women. Each woman is unique; some heal more quickly than others. The inborn strength of one person's tissues may be different from that of another. However, the likelihood of permanent nerve damage does increase with the number of babies delivered, as the tissues tend not to heal as well with each subsequent injury. The baby's size probably matters too, although not all studies have found this to be a factor. However, it makes sense that the bigger the baby or the smaller the pelvic bones, the more pressure is exerted on the pelvic muscles and nerves. Right now, there is not an accurate enough way to estimate the size of a baby or the size of the pelvic bones to warrant inducing labor before a baby is thought to be too big for the mother. We probably all know small women who have delivered large babies easily. Ultrasound can measure the size of the baby's head somewhat accurately, but it cannot tell us the size of the pelvis or how flexible the pelvis will be during labor. Therefore, obstetricians are generally unable to predict which deliveries will be difficult and which easy.

CAN CHILDBIRTH WEAKEN THE BLADDER?

Labor and delivery may stretch, strain, or even tear the muscles and the supporting tissues that hold the uterus, bladder, and rectum in their proper places. The nerves may also be stretched and injured, weakening the signals that would otherwise keep the muscles working properly. Some women suffer no damage from labor and delivery; some have damage to the nerves; some have damage to the muscles and supporting ligaments; some have damage to every one of these areas.

If injury results from a delivery, the weakened support of the bladder, rectum, or uterus may cause dropping of these organs into the vagina. Dropping of any of these organs is called *pelvic relaxation,* or *prolapse.* The muscles and supporting tissues that are above the vagina and that hold the bladder up are weakened or torn, allowing the bladder to drop down into the vagina. This bulging of the bladder into the vagina is called *bladder prolapse,* or *cystocele* (see Figure 8-1). The urethra, the tube that you urinate from, can also drop down. This combination of changes in the normal position of the bladder and urethra and weakened nerve signals may interfere with the bladder function with resulting leakage of urine (see Chapter 1).

CAN KEGEL EXERCISES DURING PREGNANCY PREVENT INCONTINENCE?

Kegel exercises, fully described in Chapter 5, help to strengthen the muscles in the pelvis. Exercising these muscles during pregnancy has been shown to decrease incontinence during pregnancy and right after delivery. A recent study evaluated two groups of women for incontinence ten months after delivery. One group had pelvic floor muscle training using a combination of Kegel exercises taught by biofeedback and mild electrical stimulation to contract the pelvic muscles (see Chapter 5) twice a week for six weeks. The other group had no such training. Twenty percent of the women who had pelvic floor training showed a decrease in incontinence ten months later, compared to only 2 percent of women who did not have the training. However, we still do not know if these exercises will prevent the development of incontinence in the years that follow.

CAN CHILDBIRTH WEAKEN THE RECTUM?

The muscle and connective tissues that hold the rectum in its place under the vagina may be weakened or torn by labor and delivery, allowing the rectum to bulge up into the vagina (see Figure 8-3). The term *rectal prolapse,* or *rectocele,* is often used by doctors to describe this change in the contour of the vagina. After delivery of a baby, some degree of prolapse is very common. However, in most women it heals and resolves within a few months without any treatment. If the problem is severe and does not resolve, some repair might need to be done.

Ellen's Story

Ellen delivered her first child, a 9-pound, 10-ounce very large bundle of joy. Getting such a large baby into the world caused quite a bit of damage to Ellen. It was obvious that she would need some stitches to fix a large tear in her vagina. While a birthing bed and room are lovely to look at and cozy to be in, they do not have the same lighting and equipment that are available in a delivery room. Ellen's obstetrician was concerned about the extent of this tear and wisely suggested moving her to where the damage could be clearly seen and repaired. Ellen and Abe, her husband, were thrilled with their son and immediately agreed to do what was necessary. Since her baby was only minutes old, the epidural anesthesia Ellen had had to ease the delivery was still working very well. She could not feel her legs at all and was oblivious to the tear. Ellen contentedly nursed her big baby, David, while being wheeled from the birthing room to the delivery room. When she needed to be moved to an operating table, the proud father escorted the baby to the nursery. Ellen's obstetrician made a wise choice. With the benefit of the operating room lights and Ellen's legs in stirrups, he could see the full extent of the injury. There was a tear right through the back wall of the vagina into the rectum. The anal muscle was completely ripped, a sure sign of a problem ahead if not treated. If Ellen had been sent home without a careful surgical repair, she would probably have needed to have surgery at some later point because of anal incontinence. With the bright lighting, effective anesthesia, and nursing assistance,

Ellen's injury was fixed. That would have been impossible if she had still been in the birthing bed. Ellen recovered quickly and left the hospital forty-eight hours later with newborn David, the infant they nicknamed "Big D."

CAN CHILDBIRTH LEAD TO ANAL INCONTINENCE?

The muscles that lie directly below the vagina and encircle the rectum are the muscles that control bowel movements. During the final phases of labor, when the baby is pushed through the vagina, these muscles are subjected to enormous forces and pressures. As a result, injury may occur. Just as for urinary incontinence, there is a higher likelihood of anal incontinence in a woman following a vaginal delivery than following a cesarean section. Studies show that more than a third of women who deliver vaginally have some damage to the anal muscles. In women who have undergone a forceps delivery, about 80 percent have damage to the anal muscles. Injured nerves can also be found in these women. Most recover their prelabor function, but for some the damaging effects can persist for years. The result of severe injury to the anal muscles and nerves can be the inability of the anal muscle to close entirely, with resultant involuntary loss of gas or stool.

Despite obstetricians' efforts to repair all apparent tears right after vaginal delivery, they can repair only what they can see, the outside anal muscle. However, much of the damage may have been done to other anal muscles, higher up in the rectum and not easily seen by the doctor. About one third of women have this type of damage. In addition, if the muscle is injured, the harm may be hidden under skin that appears normal (this is called an *occult,* or hidden, injury) and may not be visible to the doctor at all. Since these anal muscles are what give us control over the release of solid waste, failure to repair them can lead to incontinence of stool or gas (see Chapter 11). Even after repair, a few women still experience some degree of incontinence of stool or gas. That said, some women who have incomplete healing of the anal muscles do not have anal incontinence, so there must be other factors involved. Traditional methods of repair of these muscles taught to obstetricians are occasionally inadequate. We hope that with further study of how these muscles are injured, new repair techniques will help avoid incontinence.

CAN EPISIOTOMY LEAD TO ANAL INCONTINENCE?

Just before the delivery of the baby's head, an incision may be made by the doctor in the skin, and sometimes also in the muscle, in the bottom portion of the vagina to allow more room for the baby to deliver. This incision, called (midline) *episiotomy,* is supposed to avoid incidental tearing of the vagina or rectum as the baby delivers. Episiotomy is a recent practice, devised in order to substitute a straight, clean, easy-to-repair surgical incision for the jagged tear that might otherwise occur. This incision is also intended to shorten labor by giving the baby's head more room so delivery can be easier and faster. It was previously thought that faster delivery would decrease the risk of injury to the mother's bladder and would be gentler on the baby's head. However, studies have shown no evidence that these assumptions are true.

Much to everyone's surprise, episiotomy may actually cause, not prevent, pelvic prolapse and incontinence, exactly what it was supposed to help prevent. Cutting through the vaginal skin weakens this area and increases the likelihood that the skin will rip further down, possibly tearing into the anal muscle directly below the vagina. If the skin stretches naturally, it is less likely to split apart, and if it does tear, the tear is likely to be shorter. Studies have shown that episiotomy may actually lead to *more damage* of the anal muscles. If injury occurs, control of the anal muscles may be partially lost, and incontinence of gas or stool may result. For these reasons, it is probably best not to have a routine episiotomy at the time of delivery. Women need to discuss episiotomy with their doctors before the baby is due. More about anal incontinence can be found in Chapter 11.

CAN PELVIC INJURY RESULTING FROM DELIVERY BE FULLY REPAIRED?

After delivery, the doctor inspects the vagina and rectum for any tears that might have resulted from the birth of the baby. Repairs are usually made to visible cuts and tears. Unfortunately, much of the damaged tissue, the muscles, and the nerves, is covered over by the vaginal skin and is not visible to the doctor.

Recent studies, performed by ultrasound to measure these muscles right after delivery, have shown that much more damage occurs than was previously assumed. Since this is an area of concentrated research, new techniques to both recognize and repair any muscle damage should be forthcoming. We imagine that in the future obstetricians might use an ultrasound machine in the delivery room to show any postdelivery injuries to the rectum and vagina and make necessary repairs immediately. We hope this will make prolapse and incontinence less likely in the future. Currently, there are no easily available means to determine if any nerves have been damaged by a delivery, and unfortunately, there is still no way of repairing damaged nerves.

DOES CESAREAN SECTION PROTECT AGAINST PROLAPSE AND INCONTINENCE?

Because cesarean section avoids the stretching and tearing of the muscles and nerves that occur as the baby's head comes through the pelvis, it makes some sense that women who have a cesarean section might have less of a risk of urinary incontinence, anal incontinence, and pelvic prolapse. In fact, a few studies have shown just that. However, most women who deliver vaginally remain continent, so no one is proposing that all women have cesarean sections in order to avoid the possibility of later incontinence. We clearly do not understand all the factors that determine who will develop incontinence, so cesarean section is not necessary in many women with long or difficult labors. With our present understanding, many women would have to have cesareans in order to prevent one woman from developing incontinence. In addition, cesarean section has its own risks, including bleeding and the possible need for transfusion, the possibility of infection, and the risks of anesthesia and surgical injury to the bladder or intestines. The prolonged discomfort and recovery from a cesarean section at a time when the mother wants to be focused on caring for her baby are also not in anyone's best interest.

Some studies regarding deliveries and bladder health have found a number of factors that might increase the risk of developing incontinence or prolapse. These studies are based on a small sample (a relatively small number) of women, and the results show somewhat differing risk factors. However, these studies do show that a large baby, a mother with small pelvic bones, a prolonged labor, a baby whose head is in the wrong position during labor, or the use of forceps can be associated with the later development of incontinence. As further research continues to shed light on factors that contribute to incontinence, women should consider discussing potential risk factors with their obstetricians before or during labor. Multiple risk factors might convince a woman and her physician to choose a cesarean section rather than a vaginal delivery. Interestingly, one survey found that 31 percent of female obstetricians would prefer a cesarean section for themselves even if there were no problems with their pregnancy or labor. Eighty percent of these female doctors say they would make this choice in order to protect themselves from the possible development of incontinence or prolapse. Because the research is still not entirely clear, the subject of preventive cesarean section is controversial, to say the least. Only further research will determine whether obstetricians need to change the advice given to women about labor, vaginal delivery, and cesarean section.

CAN ANYTHING BE DONE TO PREVENT INCONTINENCE THAT RESULTS FROM CHILDBIRTH?

No one is advocating that all women have babies by cesarean section. While many women show evidence of injury to the muscles and nerves in the pelvis after delivery, most of the injuries heal, and most women do not go on to develop incontinence. Other factors, including the inborn strength of the body's tissues, contribute to the risk of incontinence. We do not yet know enough to predict exactly which women are at risk and therefore which women would benefit from cesarean section. However, there are some things that might be avoided in order to decrease the likelihood that pelvic injury will occur.

- The contractions of the uterus alone should be allowed to push the baby down the birth canal, without having the mother push. This has been shown to decrease the risk of injury to the nerves and muscles of the pelvis. Having the mother push the baby down the birth canal is often encouraged as soon as the cervix is fully dilated. Words of encouragement to "push, push, push" are heard in Lamaze classes and labor rooms everywhere. It appears that this may not be the best advice, however. Patience instead of pushing at this time may decrease the risk of developing incontinence. Pushing can be saved for the delivery of the baby's head.
- Although doctors now cut episiotomies in more than half of

all vaginal deliveries, this practice should be discouraged. Because episiotomies increase, rather than decrease, the risk of damage to the anal muscles, the baby's head should be allowed to come out naturally. As the baby's head descends, massaging of the area between the vagina and the rectum, called the perineum, may help gently stretch and soften the skin and underlying muscles and prevent tearing. If a tear occurs naturally, it is less likely to go through the anal muscles. In the future, as improved techniques are developed, doctors may be able to repair muscles higher in the anal canal with better results.

- Proper positioning of the mother and excellent lighting are important for the doctor to achieve the best possible repair of injured tissues and muscles. While giving birth in a birthing room is a wonderful experience, the birthing room may not be the best place to repair injuries to the vaginal muscles. Sometimes such injuries require a move to a delivery room or operating room. Proper repair should increase the strength of these tissues and muscles and decrease the risk of future incontinence and prolapse.

- The use of forceps should be discouraged. Substantial, documented evidence has shown that the use of forceps increases the risk of injury to the nerves and muscles of the pelvis, much of which is irreversible.

- A much more liberal approach to the use of cesarean section for women who have a large baby, small pelvic bones, a baby whose head is in the wrong position, or a prolonged labor may help to avoid damage to the mother. For years, obstetricians focused only on the outcome of the health of the baby at the time of delivery. Without question, this should still be their absolute priority. However, as women live longer and healthier lives, we cannot ignore the impact of difficult labors and deliveries on their long-term quality of life as well. Shortsighted obstetrical practices that ignore these problems are not in the best interest of women's health. Many women have been encouraged by doctors, nurses, childbirth educators, even friends and family to endure prolonged labors and difficult deliveries in order to have "natural" births. Most of these women are not aware of the potential risks that prolonged labor or a difficult delivery can pose to their future health and comfort.

Until recently, studies were not available for women and their doctors to show that these risks, in fact, existed. With the development of the subspecialty of urogynecology, a field of medicine dealing specifically with female incontinence and prolapse, more of this research is being performed and more widely published. As is often true, it may take years for the full effects of these findings to influence everyday obstetric practice.

Women and their doctors should discuss these issues before labor and delivery and come to some agreement as to what the reasonable choices are if labor turns out to be prolonged or difficult. Some women may choose to avoid cesarean section at all costs, while others may opt for a cesarean section early on. Don't put off having this conversation until it is too late to take an active role in the decision making. As a patient, each woman can act as both a consumer and an advocate for her own health. Being armed with information and having the courage to question will go a long way toward helping you get the best care possible.

CHAPTER 5

Treating Incontinence Without Surgery

Judy's Story

"Boy, I sure hope the next five years are better than these last five years have been," said forty-seven-year-old Judy. "First I need a cane to walk, then I go on antidepressants, and now I can't keep my pants dry! What's next?"

Judy came to our office after five rough years. Her problems had started with a serious car accident. After lots of painful physical therapy, she was now able to walk using a cane. For a while she had thought she might need a walker or wheelchair, so she was grateful for and proud of her progress. That long recuperation took its toll, though. She fell into a severe depression at one point and she needed to take antidepressants. "Things just got too hard" was how she put it. With her psychiatrist's okay, Judy stopped taking the antidepressants a few months before coming to see us. "I felt that I was really starting to get a handle on life again. I just wanted to stand entirely on my own two feet, even though one foot doesn't work so well," she said mischievously. Her sense of humor had probably helped get her through the roughest patches.

Recently, she had had episodes of profuse leaking. Her bladder would not merely leak but gush until completely empty. These were major accidents, and Judy was mortified when they occurred at work. She was the administrator for a large children's welfare agency and found the days very stressful but "good for my soul." Taking what she thought was the "easy way out" of her bladder problem, she bought larger and larger absorbent pads until she was using a large diaper-type pad with a large absorbent pad inside it. Despite full-contact padding, she had an accident at work one day that ended with urine-soaked clothes and a puddle on the floor. There was a photography darkroom nearby, and she quickly slipped inside, climbed up on the counter, sat in the sink, and rinsed off. Her clothes were now clean but very wet, so she used the blow dryer intended for photographic prints to dry off her clothes. What a story!

We all agreed that she was enormously quick-thinking and resourceful but that there had to be a better way. Her history, physical, and urodynamics evaluation gave us a complete picture. She was single and had never had children, so we weren't looking for injury from childbirth. Her pelvic exam was normal, but during the urodynamics study she had bladder spasms when her bladder was full. These spasms caused her to empty her bladder completely wherever she was when they struck. Judy was glad to hear that bladder spasms are always treated by nonsurgical means.

In a discussion with Judy's psychiatrist, we realized that we could "kill two birds with one stone" by prescribing a medicine that treats depression and also has the side effect of reducing bladder spasms. In addition to the medication, we prescribed a biofeedback program and pelvic floor exercises, all to be completed in three sessions. Judy did very well with this course of treatment. On a follow-up visit she reported that she had had no leaking and no puddles. "Maybe the next five years won't be so bad after all," she said on her way out of the office.

WHAT CAN BE DONE TO TREAT INCONTINENCE WITHOUT SURGERY?

Modern medicine gives us very effective options to treat incontinence that do not involve surgery. If you fear surgery—and honestly, we all do—be assured that a urogynecologist has a whole host of treatments available that may help you. This array of treatments includes simple changes in diet, exercises for the bladder, using a "bladder diary" to retrain your bladder, biofeedback, several easy-to-use devices, and various oral medications. The best choice of therapy depends upon the type and severity of the problem. This chapter explains these nonsurgical treatments. Use it as a starting point for discussing treatment options with your doctor so that you can find the most comfortable and effective choice for you.

CAN DRINKING TOO MUCH WATER CAUSE URGENCY AND FREQUENCY?

Allison's Story

Allison was a self-described "happy health nut." She'd read many articles in women's magazines warning of the dangers of dehydration and urging women to drink at least eight 8-ounce glasses of water each day. Allison bought herself a large water bottle with a mesh holder that she could sling over her shoulder, and she took it everywhere. She found herself drinking water at the hardware store, at the post office, in the car, at work. Water, water, everywhere. At first she happily thought about how she was "flushing all those toxins" out of her system. She envisioned her organs contentedly awash in fresh, clean bottled water. But before long, she found herself rushing to bathrooms all over town. Once she embarrassed herself as she frantically unzipped on the way into a public ladies' room and ran smack into an old flame who happened to be standing right at the entrance. When she came into the office for her regular checkup and Pap smear, she mentioned the problem.

We asked her to keep a "bladder diary," basically a record of all the fluids she drank and the amount of urine she passed for two days. After realizing she was drinking four times the amount of liquid she needed, we suggested she cut down to 32 ounces a day. Within two days, she noted a major improvement in her problem. The "bladder diary" helped us find an easy cure.

We see women in our office every day who drink water all day long and then wonder why they have to urinate all the time. Obviously, if water goes in, it has to come out! Large volumes of water will overtax all but the healthiest bladders. Drinking more than four glasses of water a day may cause your bladder to become temporarily overstretched and may lead to urgency and even incontinence. And if you already have a problem with your bladder, overtaxing it will only make the problem worse. As with everything else, use moderation when drinking water. Let your thirst be your guide.

CAN DIETARY CHANGES HELP URGENCY AND URGE INCONTINENCE?

Urgency means you frequently feel the need to urinate. There are some simple dietary changes that may give you significant relief.

In addition to the amount of fluid you drink, the kind you drink is also important. You should be aware that caffeine and alcohol act as diuretics. A diuretic forces more water out of your system than it puts in. So even a moderate amount of coffee, tea, cola, or alcohol increases the amount of urine that your bladder has to deal with, and this can lead to frequency and urgency.

Caffeine, nicotine, alcohol, spicy foods, carbonated beverages, and citrus fruits contain substances that irritate the bladder lining. When these irritants collect in the bladder, they may cause the bladder muscle to have spasms that lead to frequency, urgency, and, in some cases, incontinence. A recent study found that four or more cups of brewed caffeinated coffee a day (instant coffee has less caffeine) leads to urgency in most women; for some women just two cups can create the same problem.

If you eat or drink any of these potential irritants, experiment to see which ones might be responsible for your problem. We usually suggest eliminating all these irritants from your diet for two weeks. If the symptoms go away, introduce one thing at a time back into your diet until you identify the troublemaker. Often just avoiding the things that irritate your bladder will go a long way toward curing the problem. If, on occasion, you really want to have something that you know will irritate your bladder, be aware that you may have to stay close to a bathroom for the day.

Caffeine Content (per 5-ounce serving)

Coffee	Brewed:	140 mg
	Instant:	65 mg
	Decaf:	5 mg
Tea (black)	Brewed:	70 mg
	Instant:	30 mg
Chocolate	Dark, solid (1.5 ounces):	31 mg
	Milk, solid:	10 mg
	Milk drink:	3 mg

Beverages (per 12-ounce serving)

Coke, Diet Coke:	50 mg
Mountain Dew:	54 mg
Pepsi:	40 mg
Jolt:	72 mg
Dr Pepper:	40 mg
Sprite:	0 mg
7-Up:	0 mg

Medications

Darvon:	35 mg
Dexatrim:	200 mg
NōDōz:	100 mg
Excedrin:	65 mg
Midol:	35 mg
Dristan:	17 mg
Vanquish:	33 mg

Sources: National Coffee Association, National Soft Drink Association.

CAN EXERCISE TREAT URGENCY, URGE INCONTINENCE, OR STRESS INCONTINENCE?

The pelvic muscles help to hold the bladder and urethra in their proper places. When these muscles weaken, the bladder and urethra drop out of their normal positions and, as a result, may no longer work properly. Just as walking or jogging helps keep your legs strong and toned, exercising the pelvic muscles can help you strengthen the muscles that control urination. If you build up strong muscles, you will sometimes be able to contract them before a cough or sneeze to prevent the loss of urine. If you frequently feel the urge to urinate, try consciously contracting these muscles, as described below. This voluntary contraction triggers a reflex reaction that relaxes the bladder and stops bladder spasms, and the urge should subside temporarily. Pelvic muscle exercises can really help you control urgency and urge incontinence. Dr. Arnold Kegel first described these exercises in the late 1940s. The Kegel exercises are not difficult to do, but, like any exercise, they need to be done regularly to be really effective.

HOW CAN YOU USE KEGEL EXERCISES TO PREVENT LEAKING?

Kegel exercises can come in handy when you feel the urge to urinate. In addition to helping you strengthen the supporting pelvic muscles, a Kegel contraction can help you prevent leaking. If you have a problem with urgency incontinence, as soon as you feel the urge to urinate, contract your pelvic muscles. This voluntary contraction will trigger a reflex signal to the brain that automatically causes the bladder to relax. Then take a few deep breaths and try to relax so that anxiety doesn't trigger another spasm. With the bladder calmed down, you can take the time to find a bathroom

Many women lose urine when they shift from a sitting to a standing position. Many think stress incontinence causes this, but it is usually the result of a bladder spasm triggered by the change in position. If this happens to you, tighten the pelvic floor muscles just before you stand up. The contraction of the muscles will start the reflex that relaxes the bladder and should help prevent loss of urine. The same technique can be used for "key-in-the-door" incontinence. Sometimes just approaching the front door with a full bladder causes some women to start to leak. Tighten your pelvic muscles before you put the key in the door. You should be able to feel your bladder relax. Then release the Kegel contraction, open the door, and head to the bathroom.

You can sometimes anticipate situations that will lead to stress incontinence. If you need to lift something heavy, contract the pelvic muscles and hold them contracted during the lifting, so that the flow of urine is stopped. If you are about to cough or sneeze, even if you have just the slightest warning, there's time to tighten the pelvic muscles. Sometimes this completely eliminates incontinence. Often, simple strategies like these can be enough to control the problem and help you avoid more involved medical treatments. Pelvic floor muscles are like all other muscles—you tone them and keep them fit with regular exercise, so keep doing your Kegels!

How to Do Kegel Exercises

First, figure out which are the correct muscles by sitting on the toilet with your legs slightly apart. Start to urinate normally, but after a few seconds, without moving your legs, try to stop the stream of urine. If you are able to stop the stream of urine, you are probably using the correct muscles. If you are not able to stop the stream, keep trying. Maybe you've never tried or even thought about this before. Once you have identified the correct muscles, exercise them by tightening them for a slow count of five and then relax. However, once you have identified the muscles, don't continue to practice the exercises while you are urinating. Sometimes trying to urinate (which relaxes the sphincter muscle) and at the same time perform a Kegel (which tightens the sphincter) can confuse the bladder and cause spasms. These isometric exercises should be repeated ten times in the standing, sitting, and reclining positions, at least three times per day, for a total of ninety contractions per day. The improvement won't be immediate, but in a few weeks to few months you will likely notice an improvement.

Ninety contractions a day may sound like a lot of exercise, but this routine requires no special equipment and can be easily incorporated into your daily life. Since no one can see you exercising these muscles, you can exercise anytime and anywhere. You don't need a gym membership to do Kegels! Do your Kegel exercises while brushing your teeth, driving to work, reading the paper, or sitting at a desk. Some women get in the habit of doing Kegels at

every red light or stop sign. After a while, performing Kegels becomes automatic.

The good news is that about 70 percent of women will notice
improvement from these exercises, meaning that many women
will be able to avoid medication and/or surgery. But, like any form
of exercise, they will work only if you do them regularly. Once you
notice improvement, continue to exercise every day to maintain
the good results. It might help to make little reminders for yourself. If you do forget for a period of time, just restart your routine.
It really can and should be incorporated into your daily schedule.

There may be a bonus for you in doing these exercises. Kegel
exercises are known to improve a woman's sex life. They don't
make your partner any better-looking, but they do improve functioning of your pelvic muscles and your sexual satisfaction. Give
Kegels a try; they can truly improve the quality of your life!

Some women have trouble learning to perform Kegel exercises
properly. If that's the case for you, talk to your doctor because there
are ways he or she can help. Here are some of them.

ARE THERE OTHER NONSURGICAL DEVICES TO TREAT INCONTINENCE?

Biofeedback

Biofeedback is one tried-and-true way to help you learn the
proper way to strengthen your pelvic muscles. By the time you
reach adulthood, you don't really think about the muscles you use
to control your bladder. Consequently, many women have a hard
time isolating the muscles they need to contract in order to exercise and strengthen the pelvic floor. A trained professional can
help you learn how to contract these muscles properly. He or she
will place a special sensor in the vagina that detects muscle contractions. If the correct muscles are contracted, a line on the
sensor's monitor will get higher and higher. If the exercise is not

performed properly, the line on the monitor will not change at all. Since you are using your vision (biologic) to reinforce (feed back) the correct muscle contractions, this is a type of biofeedback.

This technique is easily and painlessly learned one on one with a trained nurse or physical therapist. In a large Norwegian study involving several thousand incontinent patients, one group of women was taught pelvic floor exercises over six months in small classes with a physical therapist while the other group performed the exercises but received no personal instruction. At the conclusion of the study, 70 percent of the women who received personal instruction were able to stay dry significantly more often than the group of women who were not in the classes.

Most of our patients get the hang of these pelvic floor exercises relatively quickly and are very proficient after just one or two forty-five-minute sessions with a trained nurse. We suggest a review session two weeks later and another one a month later to reinforce the technique. With this training, most women are able to master Kegel exercises.

We recently presented our success rates with biofeedback to AUGS, the American Urogynecological Society. This national medical society reviews results and is the scientific body disseminating information about incontinence and prolapse. We're proud to say that AUGS reviewed our five-year follow-up study of patients using the three-session biofeedback program and found the results to be in line with the national data on biofeedback success.

Jackie's Story

Jackie is a fit, trim, highly disciplined forty-nine-year-old housewife. She prides herself on her daily workouts, low-fat diet, and daily sets of Kegel exercises. "I'm determined to give old age a run for its money," she told us. "I'll go out kicking and screaming when it's my time. Until then I'm willing to work my butt off to stay healthy." She came into the office one day disappointed because, despite her Kegel exercise regime, she still had mild incontinence. We asked Jackie to demonstrate a Kegel during her physical exam. It appeared that most of her efforts were going into contracting the wrong muscles. She did the exercises regularly and diligently, but she did them incorrectly. We find that many women perform Kegels ineffectively because they don't know exactly which muscles to contract. Biofeedback to the rescue! With it, we've taught hundreds of women to gain control over their pelvic floor muscles.

Jackie spent three sessions with our incontinence nurse and the biofeedback equipment. This equipment senses the pelvic floor contraction as well as some surrounding muscle contractions. Jackie could see all of this muscle activity monitored on a screen. She then learned to isolate and contract only the targeted muscles. Now she could make all that exercising efficient and effective. We put Jackie on the three-session exercise program devised at our center. The initial teaching session was for forty-five minutes. Jackie then returned two weeks later for a tutorial and reinforcing session. We reviewed her voiding diary and the amount of fluid she was drinking each day. Four weeks later she came in for her last session. Jackie felt confident in being able to exercise correctly on her own, which we told her she would need to do indefinitely to keep her pelvic muscles well toned and strong.

Jackie made good use of the biofeedback sessions and has incorporated proper Kegel exercises into her daily routine. Every time she comes into the office she tells us she's still fighting the good fight to stay fit and healthy. "I'm dry and so grateful," she said.

The Neotonus Chair

Wouldn't it be wonderful if you could exercise without having to do anything? Well, your wish has been granted. The Neotonus chair is a way to effortlessly, painlessly, and safely exercise the muscles that support the bladder. The chair is a comfortable wood chair with a padded seat. Under the seat is an electromagnet connected to a computer. Based on a preset program, the computer turns the magnet on and off every few seconds. The magnet triggers a weak electrical impulse in the muscles of the pelvis, causing them to contract without any effort on your part. All you feel is a slight "ping" in the pelvic floor as the muscles contract and a pleasant feeling as the muscles slowly relax.

You sit on the chair fully dressed and can read a magazine or do work if you wish (Figure 5-1). No cell phones or laptops, however, because the chair's magnet would interfere with their operation. For the first ten minutes, the chair's computer stimulates the mus-

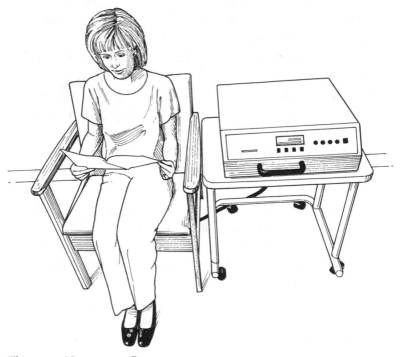

Figure 5-1: NEOTONUS CHAIR

cles holding up the pelvis. Then, for the next ten minutes, a second type of signal stimulates other muscles that are responsible for stopping the stream of urine.

Using the chair for twenty minutes twice a week for eight weeks makes a big difference in the strength of these muscles. The results have been good, with essentially no effort on the woman's part. The effects can be long-lasting, but you may have to see your doctor for a tune-up every now and then. Currently, the chairs are available at a limited number of gynecologists', urogynecologists', and urologists' offices or clinics. Because the chair is so easy to use, it may soon become an important way to help women with incontinence.

Marie's Story

Marie is an elegant seventy-four-year-old woman who loves to organize charity events and travel with her grandchildren. Each of her four oldest grandchildren has been treated to an educational tour of Europe, accompanied by their very refined and cultured grandmother.

When she came into the office, Marie complained of mild stress and urge incontinence, and we immediately sensed that pelvic floor exercises could lead to a dramatic improvement. We taught her Kegel exercises in the office, but she just "couldn't get it." When biofeedback was suggested to help her learn which muscles to contract, Marie balked. She just could not see herself undressed and working actively with a machine, even if the whole process was painless and private. She reluctantly agreed to try it, but after three canceled appointments, we knew it just wasn't going to work for her.

At about the time of her next routine physical, we had installed a Neotonus chair in our office and suggested it as a treatment option. When she heard she could sit in a comfortable chair for twenty minutes twice a week for eight weeks with no need to undress or exercise, her face lit up. "Oh, I like the sound of this. It seems like just my style," she said.

For the next eight weeks, Marie contentedly sat in the Neotonus chair reading a magazine while the magnetic stimulation exercised her muscles for her. As an extra bonus, she could feel the contractions and was able to figure out how to do proper Kegels on her own between visits. Within several months her mild incontinence was resolved, and she was happily enticing her fifth and youngest grandchild to join her on a trip to Rome and Paris.

Electrical Pelvic Muscle Stimulation

If you have had trouble figuring out the right muscles to contract or have weak pelvic muscles, here's another technique to help strengthen the pelvic muscles. Electrical pelvic muscle stimulation is not as frightening as it sounds and requires very little effort on your part. A small tube is inserted into the vagina or the rectum to deliver a tiny electrical signal that causes the pelvic muscles to contract (Figure 5-2). The signal feels like a hum in the muscle and is not at all uncomfortable. This technique can be used to start a program of pelvic floor exercise to treat either stress or urge incontinence.

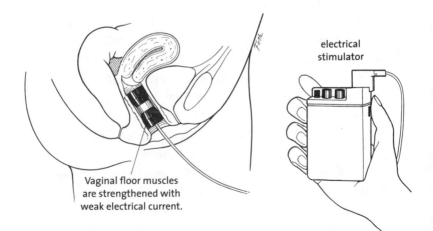

electrical
stimulator

Vaginal floor muscles
are strengthened with
weak electrical current.

Figure 5-2: PELVIC MUSCLE STIMULATOR

The electrical pelvic muscle stimulation treatment involves use of the device for fifteen to thirty minutes one or two times a day, on a schedule outlined by your doctor. Although this method is more awkward than the Neotonus chair described above, it is less expensive and can be done at home. The electrical stimulation device is small and is placed just inside the vagina, like a tampon. It is an easy way to produce noticeable improvement in muscle tone and bladder control. Your doctor should be able to order the device for you if it's not on hand in the office.

Joan's Story

"I've been lucky with multiple sclerosis, but now this little problem is really getting in my way," said fifty-five-year-old Joan when she came into our office. Joan had a mild case of multiple sclerosis that had been stable for years. Along with her MS had come a little frequency and urgency to urinate hourly during the day. Since she made her living as a piano teacher, the hourly need to urinate sometimes struck during a lesson or in midconcerto. The problem and Joan's worry grew a bit worse each year.

We spent some time trying to teach her pelvic floor exercises with biofeedback, but our nurse informed us that, in Joan, these muscles were particularly weak and would need some help before the biofeedback program could work. We decided to add electrical stimulation in the form of a device she could use at home. Each day, Joan inserted a slim probe, smaller than a tampon, into her vagina. When she turned the unit on, it generated a weak electrical signal to the probe that produced a feeling like a hum in her pelvic floor muscles. Joan felt only a mild tingle but could tell that the muscle was contracting. "Pelvic floor exercises the easy way" was how she put it.

Joan continued the biofeedback program in our office while using the electrical stimulation device every day at home. The combination of biofeedback and electrical stimulation worked; her frequency and urgency diminished. She still made frequent trips to the bathroom, but she could easily make it through an hour-long lesson.

Vaginal Cones

There is another method to help you isolate exactly the pelvic muscles that need strengthening. Made of plastic, vaginal cones look like smooth white suppositories and come in graduated weights, from less than an ounce to a few ounces (Figure 5-3). You insert a cone into the vagina like a tampon. Their smooth texture forces you to grip the pelvic muscles tightly in order to prevent the cone from falling out. The cone is used for about ten minutes at a time, two or three times a day.

You can use the cones while you are doing your daily activities, and your pelvic muscles will get a workout at the same time. The cones are easily removed at the end of each session by pulling on the attached string, and they can be quickly cleaned with soap and

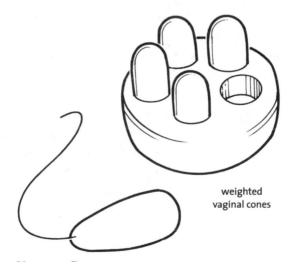

weighted
vaginal cones

Figure 5-3: VAGINAL CONES

water. You can increase the weight of the cones little by little until you regain bladder control. We sent a set of cones to a patient who had taken up residence in the desert in the Middle East, where biofeedback was not available. She found the vaginal cones helpful until she could return for a more complete treatment. The cones can also be used at home as an adjunct to biofeedback sessions. They cost less than $100 and can be ordered through your physician. Like other exercises, "workouts" with vaginal cones must be performed daily to produce a continued effect.

Sylvia's Story

In early June, Sylvia's employer—the local high school—announced that the daily schedule would change in September. The veteran Sylvia, a fifty-eight-year-old history teacher, dreaded the coming semester. For years, each class period had been fifty minutes long with a ten-minute "passing period" between classes. As part of an educational reform movement in her school district, classes were now structured in a "block schedule" of ninety minutes each. Her particular principal directed that since the students did not need the passing period to move to a different classroom, the ninety minutes should be uninterrupted instructional time. No breaks. If kids needed thirty seconds to stretch, they could do it in the classroom, but bathroom breaks should occur before and after class. Improved test scores mattered; instructional time mattered; bathroom breaks did not. The teachers as a group grumbled and moaned; Sylvia silently panicked.

Since going through menopause at forty-nine, she had found that she needed to go to the bathroom much more often. Her bladder was frequently signaling the urge to urinate. For the last few years, Sylvia had simply put her bladder on the class schedule. During each passing period, she had made a beeline for the ladies' room. Almost without fail, she had been able to urinate every fifty minutes all day long. Sylvia wasn't thrilled with her system, but it had worked—until now. The thought of having to make it through a ninety-minute period was making her very anxious. "Just thinking about standing in front of a roomful of adolescents and really needing to pee makes me feel like wetting my pants," she said. "And no way am I going to tell that dolt of a principal that I have a pee problem. Fix it, please!"

After examining Sylvia and finding everything in good shape, we realized that she had unwittingly created part of her "pee problem." When her bladder had become a bit more active at the time of menopause, she had tried to solve the problem by emptying her bladder before she really needed to go. Eventually, her bladder was signaling that it was time for a bathroom break more and more frequently. By putting herself on the fifty-minute class schedule, she had put her bladder in control. And of course her bladder was not aware when school was over, so she had this same problem at night too. Sylvia was getting up every hour or hour and a half all night long. She had grown accustomed to the interruption of work, leisure, and sleep.

We decided to give her medication to help ease the bladder overactivity and the spasms that were signaling her to go. We also recommended biofeedback to help "reprogram" her bladder. Lastly, we suggested timed voiding, so she would be able to stretch out the time between trips to the bathroom. She was greatly relieved that the "fix" was so easy. As the summer drew to a close, Sylvia was enjoying uninterrupted day trips with her friends and only one trip to the bathroom during the night. With more continuous sleep under her belt and confidence in her ability to make it through a ninety-minute period with ease, Sylvia worried only about her "dolt of a principal" as she awaited the start of a new school year.

WHAT IS TIMED VOIDING?

The average, healthy woman makes about six to eight trips to the toilet in a twenty-four-hour period, assuming a normal fluid intake of about a quart of liquid per day. Women with urinary urgency are often uncomfortable because they have the persistent sense that they need to void, even if their bladders are not full. This is distracting, distressing, and in some situations socially limiting. Many of these women plan their days around the availability of a bathroom. Other women avoid going out during the day, overnight visits, car trips, the theater, public transportation, anything that limits immediate access to a toilet. Timed voiding can help some women with this problem. Its goal is simply to help you increase the time between trips to the toilet.

Also known as *bladder drills* and *bladder training,* this technique is based on the accepted premise that bladder control is a *learned* behavior. We all began as babies in diapers with absolutely no bladder control. Back then our bladder had a mind of its own. As we grew to the ripe old age of two or three, we noticed what it felt like to have a full bladder and a wet diaper. We learned to listen to the signals telling us that we had to urinate, and we learned how to hold on until we reached the toilet.

The bladder drill is a form of behavior modification that teaches you how to regain control of when you urinate. The idea is to systematically lengthen the time between urinations according to a timed schedule. For example, if you now feel the need to urinate every hour, begin by waiting an hour and fifteen minutes between trips to the bathroom.

After a few days, this time can be increased to an hour and a half, then an hour and forty-five minutes, and then eventually to two or three hours. If you feel the urge to urinate before the allotted time, use pelvic floor contractions (Kegels), as described on page 95, to stop the bladder spasms and relieve the urge to urinate. This regimen is easy but will require that you pay attention to when you urinate for a few weeks. It is best to keep a written record of when you void in order to help you keep to the schedule. It might also help you to record your fluid intake for a bit.

While it is good to drink water during the day, the current trend of drinking quarts of water all day long may be overdone. Water that goes in has to come out. If you already have a problem with an overactive bladder, filling it rapidly won't help. Keep track of what and how much you drink. Make note of how this influences your need to go to the bathroom.

A voiding diary to keep a record of what you drink and when you urinate can be found on page 56. Make photocopies of that page, fill them out for two days, and bring them with you to your doctor or nurse to review your progress and get advice on what you can do to improve your situation. If the problem should ever occur again, you can go back to keeping a schedule until your bladder behaves again.

Often some improvement, or even a complete solution, may be apparent within the first few weeks of using this method. After your bladder relearns what it is like to be comfortably full, the longer periods between voiding will become second nature once more. In addition to bladder training, sometimes medication to control spasms can help control the frequent urge to urinate.

How Do You Keep the Timed Voiding Diary?

It is best to go over a timed voiding plan with your doctor. Reevaluation of the plan with a nurse every week or two will help determine how you are doing and make necessary adjustments. Most women find that the follow-up appointments keep them on the timed plan and give their medical professional the information to make any necessary changes in the treatment plan.

The following are general instructions for timed voiding. All you will need is a copy of the timed voiding record on page 56 and a watch.

1. Keep a record of every time you void for two days. The amount that you void is not important.
2. Figure out the *average* amount of time between trips to the bathroom for those two days.
3. Make a written plan for timed voiding by adding fifteen minutes to your *average* time between voiding.
4. The next day, empty your bladder at the scheduled time, even if you do not feel the need to go. Pelvic floor contractions (Kegels; see page 95) should be used to stop any urge to void before the scheduled time.
5. Do not void again until the next scheduled time. If you leak, don't worry about it. Stick to the written schedule of timed voiding.
6. Keep to this schedule for a week.
7. Add fifteen minutes to the time in between voiding every week until you can wait for the normal three to four hours. At this point, you, not your bladder, will be in charge of your schedule.

Maria's Story

Maria is a forty-eight-year-old high school math teacher. She came into the office reporting that she "used to have a great bladder." "I could hold my urine and go to the rest room at school just once or twice a day." Now she barely got through ninety minutes, or two classes. Since the faculty bathroom was on the other side of the building, her "new problem bladder" caused inconvenience as well as discomfort. "My students need my attention, and all I can think about is how I am going to bolt out the door at the end of class and hope I don't leak on my way as I run to the bathroom." Often the urge to go got stronger and stronger the closer she was to the bathroom, and she would leak as she closed the door of the stall and began to undress. When Maria came into our office, she was agitated and ready for a solution. "Operate on me, do anything it takes to fix this problem. I can't take it anymore!"

After doing a history and physical exam, we knew Maria had the symptoms of the onset of menopause. She had mild hot flashes and occasional night sweats. Her mother is a breast cancer survivor, and Maria told us she feared taking hormone replacement for the menopause symptoms. To complete her evaluation, we did a urine culture, checked the residual urine left in the bladder after urinating, and asked her to keep a voiding diary. It became clear that Maria suffered from an overactive bladder, a common occurrence at the onset of menopause. When the levels of estrogen start to drop in midlife, the bladder and the vagina react with drying of the vagina and urinary urgency, resulting in what we call "key-in-the-door" leakage.

The good news for Maria is that this is very treatable with pelvic floor exercises. A reflex in the spine allows the bladder to relax and stop leaking when the pelvic muscles are contracted. This skill is easily taught with the aid of biofeedback, a technique where the pelvic muscle contraction can be seen on a monitor and the woman learns to manipulate the correct muscle group while watching the screen. In our incontinence center we researched this subject and concluded that three sessions of biofeedback with daily practice of pelvic floor exercises is effective in 70 percent of women within a few months.

In addition to the biofeedback and exercises, we suggested that Maria start on vaginal estrogen tablets. Using them two nights a week at bedtime reverses the effects of thinning, drying vaginal tissues and overactive bladder. They make no mess as some creams do, and they are absorbed only minimally into the bloodstream. Maria had no reservations about the estrogen tablets and started them and the biofeedback and pelvic floor exercises immediately. After three months, she was relaxed and focused in front of her students. Helping them master algebra and geometry became her chief concern once again. "My great bladder is back!" she said.

CAN ESTROGEN IMPROVE INCONTINENCE IN POSTMENOPAUSAL WOMEN?

Both the bladder and the urethra need estrogen in order to stay healthy. Without estrogen, the cells that line the inside of the bladder and urethra become thinner and less elastic. After menopause, the ovaries make very little estrogen. After months or years without adequate amounts of estrogen, these areas generally don't function as well as they once did. Also, the lining of the bladder can become more easily irritated by substances in the diet that are filtered into the urine, such as from caffeine, alcohol, citrus fruits, carbonated beverages, or spicy foods. Therefore, menopausal women who are not taking estrogen replacement may notice a worsening of their bladder symptoms over time.

The nerves that carry signals to the bladder also need estrogen to work properly. Without estrogen the nerves may become so sensitive that you may experience urgency or have bladder spasms after even partial filling of the bladder. If this condition worsens, spasms can cause leaking. Taking estrogen allows the nerves controlling your bladder to function properly and helps prevent these spasms. Sometimes a combination of estrogen and another means of decreasing spasms, as described in this chapter, may be needed to relieve the symptoms.

Without estrogen, the blood flow to the urethral tissues decreases. Remember the image of the urethra as a doughnut? (See Figure 1-3.) With decreased blood flow, the spongy tissue around the urethra collapses, and the hole in the doughnut gets larger. As a result, more urine can slip through the urethra and leakage occurs. Estrogen increases the blood flow to the pelvic tissues, including the urethra. Normal blood flow fills the spongy tissue; the urethra stays closed, and leaking may be prevented.

Estrogen is often helpful for women with incontinence who are entering menopause or who are postmenopausal. If you start taking estrogen at the beginning of the menopause (after weighing its risks and benefits in your particular case), you may be able to avoid many of the above changes. If you have already gone through the menopause and have not taken estrogen, starting it now can often reverse the changes in the bladder and urethra and improve your symptoms. Be patient. Reversing these changes may take a few months. The use of estrogen should be discussed with your doctor in order to evaluate what is right for you. There are many ways to take estrogen, including local therapy that is limited to the bladder and vagina. These are discussed below.

WHAT IS THE BEST WAY TO TAKE ESTROGEN FOR BLADDER SYMPTOMS?

There are a number of ways to get estrogen to the tissues of the bladder and urethra. Probably the fastest way to get estrogen to these tissues is to use a vaginal cream with estrogen. The cream is inserted with an applicator at bedtime two to seven times a week, depending on how much estrogen the tissues need. Given in vaginal cream form, the estrogen's effects are focused on the vagina, bladder, and urethra. However, some of the estrogen is absorbed into the bloodstream and will reach the rest of your body. If you use an estrogen cream every day for more than a few months, you should also take progesterone to prevent overgrowth of the uterine lining cells (unless you have had a hysterectomy). With a higher dosage and daily use, estrogen in the form of a vaginal cream can afford the same protection to the heart and bones that oral estrogen does.

Another way to get estrogen to the vagina and bladder is to use an estrogen ring (Estring). The estrogen ring is a small silicone ring that is inserted in the vagina (Figure 5-4). The ring contains a very small amount of estrogen that is released slowly over ninety days. The ring can be left in place continuously and does not need to be removed for any activity, including exercise, bathing, or intercourse. Along the same lines, Vagifem is a small estrogen tablet that is easily inserted into the vagina with an applicator twice a week. The tablet sticks to the vaginal wall and releases small amounts of estrogen over a few days. With either of these methods, the dose of estrogen is low and virtually none is absorbed into the bloodstream. As a result, virtually no estrogen makes its way to the heart, bones, uterus, or other cells of the body, and no progesterone is needed to protect the uterine lining. The downside is that because the dose of estrogen is low, it may take longer to work. However, once the cells are healthy again, these methods are more convenient to use than the cream.

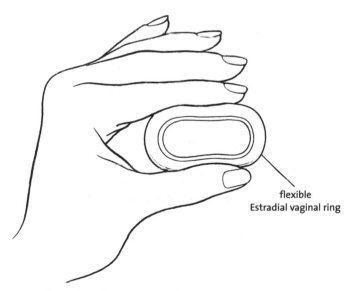

flexible
Estradial vaginal ring

Figure 5-4: ESTROGEN RING

Estrogen is also available in pill or patch form. This form of estrogen is delivered to the bloodstream and then makes its way to the bladder, vagina, and urethra. It may take longer to see positive results with this approach. If you take estrogen in pill or patch form, unless you've had a hysterectomy, your doctor should also prescribe progesterone to prevent overgrowth (or very rarely even precancerous or cancerous growths) of the uterine lining.

If you are already showing the effect of low estrogen levels—thin, pale tissue in the vagina—we usually suggest you start with the estrogen cream. If, after about six weeks, the vagina starts showing the positive effects of the estrogen, you can switch to one of the other choices. In one form or another, most women benefit from estrogen. It is best to discuss the form and dose with your doctor to establish the best option for you.

Eve's Story

Eve is a seventy-nine-year-old woman who recently married after fifteen years of widowhood. Despite her daughter Sarah's frequent entreaties over the years, Eve refused to take estrogen. "My mother didn't take any of that stuff, and I won't either!" was her attitude. "I don't like taking pills, and I won't take estrogen. I'm stubborn, and I'm old-fashioned!" she said. And she was! Years earlier Eve had actually agreed to try estrogen after Sarah had read an article about how estrogen can prevent brittle bones. But the dose was probably incorrect, since Eve began to suffer from bothersome breast tenderness after just a few weeks. Since she hadn't wanted to take estrogen to begin with, she just stopped. "I even switched doctors so I didn't have to hear about it," Eve said. "I hate taking pills!"

But now the situation had changed. Eve, a seventy-nine-year-old newlywed, was embarrassed about her urge incontinence and vaginal dryness. Her last bone density test had also showed some osteoporosis. Because of these problems, she was ready and willing to take estrogen. "Okay, Doc," she said, "I guess I'll try what you and Sarah think is best." To help Eve avoid taking too many pills, we prescribed a twice-a-week vaginal estrogen tablet for her. Eve also began biofeedback in our office to learn to do pelvic floor exercises effectively. Since she also needed something to help strengthen her bones, she reluctantly agreed to take oral estrogen as well.

Six months after her initial visit, Eve's "stubborn and old-fashioned" stance had softened. The incontinence and vaginal dryness had improved with the vaginal estrogen tablets and biofeedback training, and taking medication for her bones made her feel more confident about the years ahead. "I was a foolish old coot," she said. "Thanks for showing me a better way."

CAN MEDICATIONS BE USED TO TREAT INCONTINENCE?

There are medications available to treat stress, urge, mixed, and overflow incontinence. Different drugs affect the bladder and bladder symptoms in varying ways. Some medications relax the bladder muscle and reduce the spasms that can cause accidents. Others increase the strength of the urethral muscle and keep the bladder closed during coughing or sneezing. In general, medication alone can successfully treat about half of women with incontinence. However, medication can also be used in conjunction with estrogen, exercises, or bladder drills, which can enhance its effectiveness. Let's look at how to use medications most effectively.

Can Medications Be Used to Treat Urgency Incontinence?
Medications are available that block the spasms of an overactive bladder and can reduce or prevent urgency or urgency incontinence. Although an overactive bladder is a chronic condition,

medication may be needed only until bladder training or biofeedback helps control the problem. Urgency incontinence can often be treated with just a small dose of one of several medications. Some of the oral medications that are used for urgency incontinence are oxybutynin (Ditropan), imipramine (Tofranil), hyoscyamine (Levsin), and tolterodine (Detrol). As with most medications, there are some possible side effects. All may cause dry mouth, dry skin, constipation, or blurry vision. If these side effects occur, the dose of medication can be lowered. Tolterodine, a newer medication, is very effective and may produce fewer side effects. Both tolterodine and oxybutynin are now available in once-a-day doses, which makes taking the medication easier.

There are other medications—imipramine and doxepin are examples—that not only reduce bladder spasms but also help keep the muscles in the urethra closed. They were initially prescribed in high doses to combat depression, but by chance researchers discovered that low doses of the same medication often helped with urgency incontinence. There is no connection between depression and urgency incontinence; the medications simply seem to help both.

These medications can be used alone or in combination, depending on individual circumstances. All require a prescription and medical supervision, so you should discuss their use with your doctor. Newer medications are being developed all the time, and it is a good idea to ask your doctor about what might be newly available to help you.

Can Medications Be Used to Treat Stress Incontinence?

Stress incontinence occurs when the muscles around the urethra (sphincter) do not stay sufficiently closed, especially when you cough or sneeze (see Chapter 1). Therefore, drugs that help keep the sphincter closed can sometimes prevent urinary loss. Interestingly, these drugs are found in some common decongestants, such as Sudafed. Many women do try pseudoephedrine (Sudafed) for occasional bad days, but most cannot tolerate it daily because of the side effects of dry mouth and headache. In rare cases, these decongestants may also cause increased blood pressure or rapid heartbeat. Avoid them if you have high blood pressure. Other similar and frequently used drugs for stress incontinence are phenylpropanolamine (Ornade, Dimetapp), which are prescription drugs and must be supervised by your doctor. If you are postmenopausal, using estrogen in combination with these medications may help improve their effectiveness.

What Medications Can Be Used to Treat Mixed Incontinence?

Mixed incontinence is a combination of urgency incontinence and stress incontinence. The bladder wall has spasms, and the sphincter muscles are weak and cannot prevent leaking. Thus, this type of incontinence requires a dual solution in the form of a combination of the types of medications described above. A drug that relaxes the bladder wall muscle is used in conjunction with a drug that keeps the bladder sphincter closed. Estrogen is also usually added in postmenopausal women to keep the tissues more elastic and healthier.

Can Medications Be Used to Treat Overflow Incontinence?

Remember that overflow incontinence results when you are unable to empty your bladder fully and the urine continues to fill the bladder until it overflows and spills out. This problem can sometimes be treated with drugs that relax the urethral sphincter and allow the urine to pass more freely. Other medications, such as bethanechol, may be used to encourage the bladder to contract and force the urine out. These medications, however, are not very effective, and self-catheterization (see page 121) may be necessary.

What Are the Side Effects of These Medications?

With some medications, there may be side effects. The likelihood of getting side effects is sometimes related to the amount or kind of medication taken. When medication is taken in small doses, the side effects are generally negligible. Some medications may cause dry mouth, dry skin, nausea, or constipation. In rare cases, patients may experience blurred vision, slight confusion, or dizziness. Side effects may differ from one medication to another; therefore, changing medications may eliminate any problems. The goal, then, is to work with your doctor to get the proper dose of the right medication to help you, while avoiding particular medications or dosages that result in vexing side effects. It is very important to let your doctor know about any other medications you may be taking for other medical problems. Drugs can interact with each other, changing the effectiveness of one or both. Additionally, the combination could lead to more severe side effects. You should also tell your doctor about any other medical problems you have. For example, some of the drugs prescribed for incontinence may worsen glaucoma.

CAN MEDICATIONS FOR OTHER MEDICAL CONDITIONS LEAD TO INCONTINENCE?

Once again, it is important to tell your doctor all the medications you are taking. Some drugs can actually *cause* incontinence. For example, some antidepressants can cause urinary frequency; some of the medications used to treat urgency can make it difficult to empty your bladder; and other antidepressants may cause incontinence. Adjusting the dose of your medication or changing to another medication may be the only thing you need to do in order to relieve your symptoms. Of course, any change in medication should be discussed with the doctor who prescribed it in the first place.

WHAT IF I'M INCONTINENT ONLY WHEN I EXERCISE?

Lynne's Story

Lynne, a forty-five-year-old, felt she and her sons needed something fun to do together. Since she knew that the whole family was lacking in any type of self-defense skills, she thought it would be a good idea to take a martial arts class together. "I thought it was the perfect thing for us— we'd be doing it together, my kids would learn how to defend themselves, and we'd all probably get in shape."

Lynne exercised regularly, so she didn't worry about keeping up with her sons. But unlike her regular swimming, walking, and hiking, this class began with a warm-up routine with lots of jumping. "They jumped forward; they jumped backward; they jumped and then kicked; they jumped and then punched. I felt this warm gush and knew the only defending I was going to do that evening was to defend myself against humiliation and embarrassment. I'd wet my pants! That never happened before!" Lynne dropped out of the class and headed to our office for a solution.

Some women have an incontinence problem only when they are very active, for example during jogging, aerobics, or strenuous work. During normal activity, they are dry and comfortable. There are a number of ways of providing bladder support at times and occasions that can be anticipated. One method is with a device called the Introl. It comes in different sizes and is fitted by your doctor. The Introl is a ring-shaped silicon object that has two dull prongs. It is placed inside the vagina, and the prongs fit comfortably right under the urethra and hold it up. During stressful physical activity, this device keeps the urethra from moving up and down and prevents leaking. After the activity is over, you can easily remove the Introl, wash it with warm water, and put it away until it is needed again. The Introl is also an excellent idea for women who need surgery for incontinence but plan another pregnancy and don't want to have surgery until they are finished having children.

Women who wish to delay surgery for other reasons or avoid surgery altogether may also choose to use the Introl. It is also a good solution for women who have such an infrequent or minor problem that they are not interested in any of the more involved treatments. In the case of Lynne and her self-defense class, she was fitted for an Introl and used it only for the self-defense class, the only occasion where leaking occurred. Some women figure out on their own how to use a tampon much like the Introl to support the bladder during active times. Inserting a tampon before rigorous exercise might make many women feel more comfortable about staying dry. This can also work well and may be worth a try before being fitted for an Introl.

WHAT ARE OCCLUSIVE DEVICES?

Some women do not respond to medicines, devices, or exercises but are not interested in surgery. For these women, patches are available that can be placed directly over the urethra, blocking the flow of urine and preventing incontinence. One such patch, called FemAssist (produced by Insight Medical Corp., Boston, Mass.), is a soft plastic suction cup that fits over the urethra and prevents leakage. It can be used for a few hours, just when it is needed. For women who need protection only when they are exercising or hiking, this patch may be sufficient. For women who don't mind wearing pads in the house but want to avoid them while they are outside, the patch may be the answer.

WHAT IF YOU CAN'T EMPTY YOUR BLADDER AT ALL?

Although it happens very rarely, some women are unable to empty their bladders at all. In some cases this happens because the bladder or the bladder nerves are not working. In others, the urethra is partially blocked and the urine cannot pass through. Luckily, there is a simple technique, known as self-catheterization, to solve this problem. While sitting on the toilet, you wipe the urethra with water. Then you painlessly insert a very small, disposable tube called a catheter into the urethra to empty the bladder. The urine is passed directly into the toilet. This technique may be safely performed as often during the day as required. Since the catheters are small, they can easily be carried around in a purse. While this technique doesn't exactly sound appealing, it is easily learned, very effective, and well accepted by women who may have few other choices available to them.

Tina's Story

Tina was a thirty-year-old journalist born in Southeast Asia. She came to America as a teenager and did brilliantly in school. She told us, "I came to America a stranger but thrived here. I owe this country so much." Always interested in writing, she now was a freelancer who was published in some of the most popular magazines. Although she felt energetic and healthy, over time it had become increasingly hard for her to empty her bladder.

As she explained her medical history, she surprised us by mentioning that she had first noted trouble emptying her bladder starting around age twenty. Some days she would not even feel the urge to go and would need to remind herself to urinate once or twice a day. The stream of urine was slow, but she had thought nothing of it. She married in her mid-twenties, had a daughter, and continued her writing career. When she first came in to consult us at the age of twenty-eight, she also had prolapse of the uterus.

A complete workup showed that she had a huge bladder capacity; her bladder could hold a quart of urine, and she wouldn't even feel it. When she did urinate, she emptied only half of this volume and generally walked around with what for most of us would feel like a full bladder. This was a situation similar to what we call overflow incontinence, but Tina rarely leaked.

We concluded that there must be something wrong with the nerves to Tina's bladder, so we referred her to a neurosurgeon for an evaluation. He diagnosed a birth defect in Tina's spinal cord that she was not aware of, called spina bifida occulta. He predicted that this birth defect would cause more problems as Tina got older unless it was corrected with surgery. He was able to repair the birth defect, knowing that surgery would not improve her existing problems but would help ensure that she would not get worse. Since we knew the surgery would not help her empty her bladder, we taught Tina to pass a small tube through her urethra into her bladder to empty it. Tina found this easy to do, and without the weight of all that urine in her bladder, her prolapse improved.

One of the lessons we learned as a result of treating Tina was that sometimes problems elsewhere in the body actually show up first as bladder problems.

IN SUMMARY

Today we have many nonsurgical methods available to treat incontinence. What works for one woman may not work for another. The first step toward finding a solution is discussing the alternatives with your doctor. If one method fails, you may wish to try another. We have every reason to believe that you will be able to find one treatment, or a combination of treatments, that works for you.

CHAPTER 6

Treating Incontinence with Surgery

CAN SURGERY BE USED TO TREAT INCONTINENCE?

Some women try medications and exercises for relief of incontinence but are still plagued by bothersome symptoms. For these women, surgery may provide much-needed relief. Surgery is most effective when stress incontinence is a major part of the problem, and it may help if some urgency accompanies stress incontinence. It is not likely to be effective for pure urgency or urgency incontinence.

One of the goals of surgery for the treatment of incontinence is restoring the bladder and urethra to their normal position. Most women who have given birth vaginally have some degree of loosening, stretching, and even tearing of the supporting ligaments of the vagina, bladder, and rectum (see Chapter 4). This weakening of the supporting ligaments usually begins unnoticed and without any symptoms and remains that way for the majority of women for their entire lives. But for some women, the changes that occur as a result of the lengthening and stretching cause significant incontinence that interferes with their daily lives. Incontinence never jeopardizes a woman's health, but it does play havoc with a woman's ability to live life to its fullest. For those women, surgery can restore a sense of basic good health and return them to a life free of worry and wetness.

WHAT KINDS OF SURGERY CAN TREAT STRESS INCONTINENCE?

As described in Chapter 1, stress incontinence occurs when the normal support structures of the pelvic organs weaken to the point where the positions of the bladder and urethra change when you laugh, cough, or sneeze. Any number of other activities can cause leaking too. This weakness allows the force of a cough to push urine out of the bladder. If bladder tests show that you have stress incontinence, a surgical procedure can be used to help hold the urethra and bladder in the correct alignment and prevent the loss of urine.

WHAT IS AN ABDOMINAL BLADDER SUSPENSION?

The typical way to correct the position of the urethra and bladder is with an operation known as an *abdominal bladder suspension*. This operation pulls the bladder and urethra back to a normal position, supported behind the pubic bone, and holds them there. The surgery is done through an abdominal, bikini-type incision. The tissue around the urethra and near the bladder opening is stitched to the ligaments attached to the pubic bone (Figure 6-1). This operation is called a *Burch procedure,* named after the doctor who developed it.

Another variation of this procedure is called a *Marshall-Marchetti-Krantz* (MMK) *procedure,* named after the three doctors who developed this operation. With this procedure, rather than placing the stitches into the ligament, the stitches are placed di-

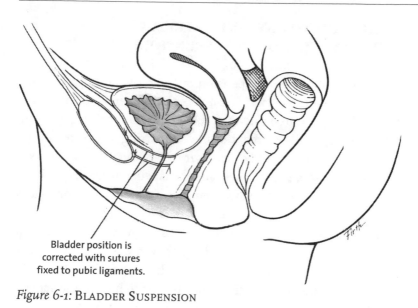

Bladder position is
corrected with sutures
fixed to pubic ligaments.

Figure 6-1: BLADDER SUSPENSION

rectly into the covering of the pubic bone. However, in rare cases, a difficult-to-treat inflammation or even an infection may occur where the sutures are placed into the bone. This problem does not occur with the Burch procedure. So while some gynecologists successfully use the MMK procedure, most gynecologists now prefer the Burch procedure to correct stress incontinence.

With either the Burch or MMK abdominal suspension procedure, the sutures are fixed to a solid object and stay in one place. This security and immobility make these repairs strong and long-lasting. The long-term (five-year) success rate for curing incontinence with an abdominal bladder suspension procedure is excellent, about 80 percent.

WHAT IS RECOVERY LIKE AFTER AN
ABDOMINAL BLADDER SUSPENSION?

An abdominal bladder suspension operation is performed in the hospital with anesthesia, either epidural or general (that is, you're put to sleep). We often find that, in addition to repairing the bladder, other reparative surgery of the supporting structures of the vagina and rectum may be necessary. Happily, it can all be performed at the same time. The bladder suspension procedure itself takes about one hour. Most women spend about two to three days in the hospital, usually because they need pain medication to help with the discomfort from the bikini incision. Most doctors leave a catheter in the bladder for a few days, or even weeks, after surgery to help drain the bladder until you are able to urinate easily.

Since the abdominal incision needs time to heal, some activity is restricted. For the first week, you can get up for meals, go to the bathroom, and take short walks. You will be fatigued, and simple activities will make you tired. After the first week you will feel stronger, be able to take longer walks, and need less rest. After about two weeks, some women begin working again from home. A few who can't avoid it go to work for a few hours a day. It takes about six weeks for most of the healing to take place. Most doctors recommend that you not do any exercise or lift anything heavier than 15 pounds for three months. This allows the formation of strong scar tissue that will hold the bladder in the proper position. After surgery, you probably should *never* lift anything heavier than 25 pounds. You don't want the force of lifting to stretch and weaken the repair work.

WHAT IS A LAPAROSCOPIC BLADDER SUSPENSION?

A laparoscopic bladder suspension technique, akin to the Burch procedure, was devised in the early 1990s. The goal of laparoscopic bladder surgery is to perform the same operation with laparoscopic instruments as would be performed with standard abdominal surgery. The laparoscopic Burch is performed through small incisions and has the advantages of less postoperative discomfort and a faster recovery. However, the procedure requires special training and skills on the part of your doctor, and not all gynecologists perform it. The laparoscope is a small telescope that is passed through a $^1/_2$-inch incision in the navel (Figure 6-2). Two or three smaller ($^1/_4$-inch) incisions are made above the pubic hairline and the operating instruments are placed through these incisions. The telescope and operating instruments are placed into the space around the bladder and specialized instruments are used to place the sutures to suspend the bladder to the ligaments near the pubic bone, just as in the Burch procedure.

The use of the laparoscope with this operation is relatively new, so long-term success rates are not yet available. However, a well-planned American study found that the success rate after five years

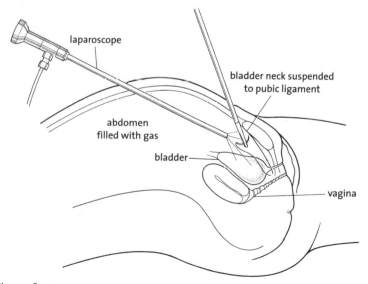

Figure 6-2: LAPAROSCOPIC BLADDER SUSPENSION

was 90 percent, just as good as that for the abdominal suspension procedures.

The laparoscopic bladder suspension operation takes about one and a half hours. It is performed under general anesthesia in a hospital or outpatient surgery center. It is very likely that with the encouraging information about success rates being published and more gynecologists being trained to perform laparoscopic bladder suspension, the procedure will become more widely available.

Dina's Story

"Okay, gang, I'm back, and I really need help," Dina said when she came in for an appointment. Dina, a sales rep, had come to our practice for many years but five years ago had moved about fifty miles away and started seeing a doctor closer to her new home. She was now in her mid-forties, with a fourteen-year-old son and a sixteen-year-old daughter. Her boy, Chris, is six feet two and weighs 180 pounds, and because he's only fourteen, she figures he has a long way to go. "I grow them really big, don't I?" she said, laughing. "Teenagers! They give me so much trouble, but I love them both to death. It's my bladder that's making me miserable." We chatted about the challenges and joys of having teenagers and then got to the sobering reason she'd come to see us.

Both of her babies had been large at birth, and the deliveries had led to some minor urinary leakage. For close to fifteen years, the incontinence had been manageable, but she had recently had a recurrence of childhood asthma and was wheezing and coughing daily. Dina thought her allergist was helping her, but he told her she would always have some wheezing and coughing despite treatment. She didn't like wheezing, but the coughing invariably left her with wet pants. "Every time I cough, I leak. On the days my allergies kick up, I might as well just stay home. I'm wet all the time," said Dina with some anxiety. On a bad allergy day, she needed to change absorbent pads four to five times. She often felt damp, itchy, and worried about odor.

Dina remembered how well we had communicated in the past and had made the hour-long drive from her new home to have us evaluate this new, embarrassing problem. The only time Dina leaked was with a cough or sneeze. She did not have to urinate frequently and did not feel a strong urge when she needed to urinate. She underwent urodynamics testing, which revealed typical stress incontinence. We could see that the amount of leakage was significant. The test showed that her bladder sphincter was working well. Her biggest problem was that the bladder neck and urethra moved a lot during the workouts her asthma and chronic cough were giving her. We wanted to put the bladder and urethra back in the proper place with something sturdy that would remain effective over the years despite the cough. Dina was looking for a relatively short recovery period. "I can't be lying around resting with two big teenagers to feed," she told us. "I need to get back to work as soon as possible."

We recommended a laparoscopic Burch procedure. It would provide support for her bladder and urethra and eliminate the incontinence, and she could be up and about in a day or two. Dina thought it sounded fine, and we proceeded with the surgery several weeks later. The bad news is that she still wheezes and coughs. The good news is that she is now dry and comfortable.

WHAT IS RECOVERY LIKE AFTER A LAPAROSCOPIC BURCH PROCEDURE?

Most women can go home the same day they have the laparoscopic Burch procedure. Since the incisions are small, there is minimal pain, and you can be up walking within a few hours. Most women do not require a catheter in the bladder and can urinate by themselves right after surgery. You can be back to most normal activities within seven to ten days. However, as with all bladder operations, you will need to allow the sutures to heal and scar tissue to form so that the repair work will hold. This takes three months, so you shouldn't do any strenuous exercise or heavy lifting (more than 15 pounds) during that time.

Emily's Story

"A lot of my friends cry about being empty nesters, but I honestly can't wait until the kids are gone. My eighth-grade son is giving me more trouble than my two daughters did together. It will be a glorious day when he matures and leaves home. I hope I live long enough to see it," Emily told us. She is a forty-three-year-old preschool teacher with three almost-grown children. Her older daughter is a junior in college; her younger daughter just began her freshman year at the state university; and her youngest child, a son, is in middle school. With only one at home right now, Emily assumed she'd be able to devote more time to taking care of herself.

For their wedding anniversary, Emily's husband, Glenn, had given her a weekly session with a personal trainer. "It seemed like the perfect gift," she said, "until I tried to use it." Vigorous exercise, she was dismayed to discover, caused quite a bit of urinary leaking. She started wearing heavier and larger absorbent pads, but their bulk irritated her. For more than a year, Emily put off getting medical help. "I just really did not want a big operation," she said. Finally the bulky pads became intolerable, and Emily made an appointment to see us.

During the exam, we had Emily cough several times, and this "stress test" was very positive. Emily had lots of leakage. Off she went to our Continence Center for a more complex but painless urodynamic test that demonstrated exactly what her bladder was doing when she leaked.

The results showed that Emily would be helped by a bladder suspension, and that it could be performed through the laparoscope. We gave Emily a quick lesson in laparoscopic bladder suspension. She learned that this is a minimally invasive method of surgery involving small ½-inch incisions made at the navel and one or two ¼-inch incisions in the mid-lower abdomen. She would be discharged within twenty-four hours and ready to drive in four to five days. She would need to restrict only one activity: she could lift no more than 15 pounds for the next three months, no matter how good she felt. Otherwise she would be able to return to her normal life. No catheter would be needed after this surgery. We counseled her that she would feel very fatigued after the surgery, even though she would have only minimal pain. Just healing from an operation takes a lot of energy. When she heard all of this, she breathed a huge sigh of relief. "I thought I'd have to be in the hospital for a week and have a long recovery with a surgery like this," she said. "Gee, now I wish I hadn't waited a year. This is a dream come true."

Her surgery went well, and Emily now enjoys her workouts with the personal trainer. For the three months following the surgery, we told Emily to avoid lifting anything heavier than 15 pounds, and these restrictions had absolutely no effect on her life. "When one of the kids at preschool wants to be picked up, I just say, 'How about a big hug instead?' Works every time."

WHAT IS A SLING PROCEDURE?

The sling procedure takes a different approach to preventing incontinence. This procedure places supporting material directly under the urethra and attaches it to the connective tissue (fascia) of the abdominal muscles. There are many variations of this operation; some doctors prefer to attach the supporting material to the ligaments near the pubic bone. The supporting material rests under the urethra like a firm hammock. When a cough or sneeze pushes the urethra down, it's forced against the sling, and the urethra is closed off. The sling procedure is often used for women who have had previous incontinence surgery that failed because of excess scar tissue formation (see Chapter 1). It is also recommended for women with a weakened urethral sphincter that does not close properly, especially when the urethra moves a lot with straining.

The surgery starts with a small incision made in the vagina, just below the urethra. Small tunnels (about $1/2$ inch wide) are then made in the connective tissue on either side of the urethra and into the space just behind the pubic bone. The sling is placed under the urethra at this point, and the ends of the hammock are brought up to the connective tissue on top of the abdominal muscles and fastened. There are a number of materials that can be used to make the sling. Some doctors prefer to use a synthetic, nylonlike material, while others choose fascia, the strong tissue that surrounds muscle, either removed from the patient or sterilized, irradiated fascia from a cadaver donor.

The success rate of the sling is very good but, like that of most incontinence procedures, not perfect. The long-term (5-year) success rate is about 85 percent. One potential, but relatively uncommon, problem with this surgery is that the sling may compress the urethra too much and block the flow of urine. Although this is rare, a small incision under the urethra can be made and one side of the sling can be cut. This usually gives the urethra more room and solves the problem. Another rare problem may develop if the urethra is blocked too much. The bladder may become overactive. Often this problem can be controlled with medication. Most women have no problems following a sling procedure; those who do still feel much better than before they had surgery, when they were frequently incontinent.

WHAT IS RECOVERY LIKE AFTER A SLING PROCEDURE?

Since the sling procedure is performed through the vagina, recovery is relatively short and there is little discomfort. Some women have some temporary swelling that presses on the urethra, and they may need a catheter for one to two weeks until the swelling goes down. Usually the patient is up and around the day after surgery and can start walking immediately. As with *all* incontinence surgery, it is important to let the sutures heal completely, which takes about twelve weeks. So for three months you should not lift anything heavier than about 15 pounds.

WHAT IS TVT?

The tension-free vaginal tape (TVT) procedure is a new procedure first developed in Sweden in 1995. This procedure is similar to the sling in principle—it forms a hammock under the urethra that bolsters it when you laugh, cough, exercise, or strain in any other way.

This procedure has been performed on more than 200,000 women in Europe and 50,000 in the United States, and the initial results are excellent. The success rate so far is 85 percent after five years. The surgery takes about thirty minutes and may be performed with local or epidural anesthesia. Most women can leave the hospital within a few hours. Patients can urinate without problems immediately after surgery.

A thin strip of supporting tape is used to form a hammock under the urethra (Figure 6-3). The tape is made of a synthetic

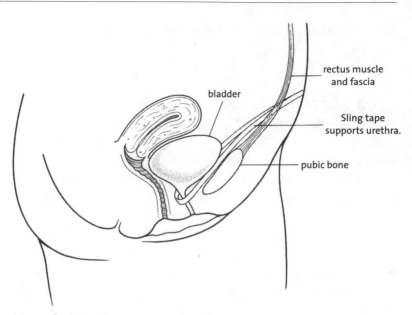

Figure 6-3: TVT PROCEDURE

nylonlike mesh that grips the surrounding tissues and holds itself in place without sutures until scar tissue grows into the mesh. Like the sling procedure, this procedure is performed through a small incision in the vagina directly below the urethra. A loose hammock is created beneath the urethra, and the ends of the hammock are pulled up through two very small ($1/2$-inch) incisions made side by side in the skin just above the pubic bone. The tape is carried up to the abdominal wall with an instrument that avoids the need for the surgeon to make a tunnel. It's faster and easier to perform than the sling procedure. Once the tape is placed properly below the urethra, the extra material is trimmed, and the incisions on the skin's surface are closed.

Because the procedure is new, the long-term (5- to 10-year) outcomes and risks are still being determined, but the results to date have been excellent. While the TVT was initially developed for stress incontinence, it has also been used with some success for

ISD combined with stress incontinence. It is likely that this procedure will be useful for many women with incontinence, and we have been impressed with the results in our own practice.

WHAT IS THE RECOVERY LIKE AFTER TVT?

Recovery following TVT is very rapid. The small incisions—the one in the vagina and the two above the pubic bone—cause only mild discomfort for a few days. Since the surgery can be performed under local or epidural anesthesia with mild sedation, there is none of the grogginess people sometimes feel after general anesthesia. Patients are usually walking around within a few hours and go home from the hospital shortly thereafter. However, as is true with all incontinence surgery, it is important to limit strenuous activity for three months to allow all the healing to take place.

Audrey's Story

Audrey has her dream job. She's an editor of a national magazine and gets to travel to exotic locations for photo shoots. "I got this job at a perfect time. My kids are grown, and I'm able to travel and see my three grandchildren anytime I want. I'm so happy with the way my life is going," she told us. But the inconvenience of packing for her last trip—to Morocco to supervise an article on North African travel—had been a wake-up call to get help with her incontinence.

The Morocco trip was for a full week, a bit longer than usual for her. She packed her large carry-on suitcase with all the clothes and toiletries she'd need for the week. But it took an entire second suitcase just to hold her supply of absorbent pads. "This is just ridiculous," she said. "At the rate I'm going, by next year I'll need a third suitcase for even more pads. I hate this!"

Audrey, who is fifty-three, first noticed mild incontinence

shortly after menopause began. She started taking oral hormone replacement plus vaginal estrogen cream, and that helped for about two years. Then her symptoms returned. We suggested biofeedback training to help her properly perform Kegel exercises. The daily pelvic floor exercises plus the hormone replacement worked well, and Audrey remained dry for about a year. Then she noticed some leaking when she coughed, sneezed, or ran. This time, greater diligence in performing the Kegel exercises had no effect, and as the problem grew, so did her supply of absorbent pads. Audrey came back in to see what her options were.

Her evaluation included a detailed history and physical exam. She also went through a urodynamic evaluation. "Those tests were almost like the biofeedback sessions I used to go to. Peeing in a commode was a little awkward, but so far getting this evaluation is a piece of cake," she told us. When we did a "leak point pressure test" by asking Audrey to bear down as though she were giving birth, she leaked quite a bit at low pressures. This told us that her urethral sphincter muscles weren't keeping her bladder closed very well. Audrey's incontinence was due to intrinsic sphincter deficiency (ISD).

Audrey had two choices: either we could inject collagen to help keep the bladder sphincter closed, or we could perform a sling surgery. After talking it over, Audrey chose surgery. "I want to fix this once and for all, otherwise I'll be too insecure to travel." Audrey's bladder needed extra support placed under the urethra. Together we decided that the TVT sling seemed the best choice. We all wanted long-term success and liked the permanent nature of TVT. The surgical procedure involves small incisions, each closed by a single stitch. Just as she hoped, the procedure involved no hospital stay.

We performed Audrey's surgery, and her stay at the outpatient surgery center was a mere six hours. She went home comfortable, urinating normally with no need for a catheter. For three days she needed mild pain medication, and then she was back in her office. She came in for her two-week checkup on a Wednesday and the next morning left for Italy to supervise an article on Tuscan villas—with only a small carry-on. Her days of absorbent pads were over.

WHAT IS AN ANTERIOR REPAIR?

An anterior, or cystocele, repair was one of the first operations developed to support the bladder and urethra to prevent incontinence. The operation supports the bladder from underneath but does not correct the loss of support experienced with the extra pressure of a cough or exercise. The anterior repair is performed through a vaginal incision just under the bladder and uses stitches to pull the strong vaginal tissue together for support. This restores the bladder and urethra closer to their original positions. Unfortunately, this operation does not work very well for incontinence, with only 37 percent of women having long-term (five-year) cures. Many doctors still use this operation for incontinence even though it is no longer state of the art. An anterior repair is a very good procedure for putting a dropped bladder back into place to relieve bulging of the bladder (see cystocele, Chapter 8). It is also helpful for women who are unable to empty their bladder because of the urine that collects in the bulging portion. But if leakage is a problem, we perform a bladder suspension operation, sling procedure, or TVT in order to successfully treat stress incontinence.

WHAT IS A VAGINAL BLADDER SUSPENSION?

This operation was designed as an alternative to the abdominal suspension. It uses sutures to hoist the bladder and urethra back up to a more normal position by attaching the sutures to strong fascia above the abdominal muscles. As the name suggests, the operation is performed through an incision in the vagina, rather than the abdomen. A small vaginal incision is made around the urethra, exposing its supporting tissues. Through this vaginal incision, stitches are placed in the supporting tissue (the fascia) next to the bladder and urethra. The ends of these long sutures are then threaded through the end of a long, narrow instrument and pulled back through a small (1-inch) incision over the pubic bone. The sutures are then tied to the layer of strong fascia on top of the abdominal muscles.

Whereas the Burch procedure attaches the urethra to an immovable pubic ligament, most vaginal suspension operations attach the urethra to connective tissue and muscles that move when you move and therefore can stretch or break the sutures. Stretching can loosen the repair work and make the surgery less effective over time. For that reason this operation is less effective over the long run, with cure rates in the 45 percent range after five years. Although some doctors still perform this procedure, we have eliminated it in our own practice because it is not effective over time.

WHAT IS RECOVERY LIKE AFTER
A VAGINAL BLADDER SUSPENSION?

Because this procedure doesn't involve a large abdominal incision, recovery is quicker and less painful than with an abdominal suspension. Surgery is also shorter, lasting about forty minutes. This operation may be a reasonable choice for some women, especially older, frailer women who might benefit from a quicker recovery. There is less discomfort because the vaginal incision is small and the abdominal incision is very small. There can be slightly more swelling around the urethra immediately after this operation, so often a catheter is left in place to drain the bladder for a few days or up to a few weeks.

Most women spend one night in the hospital after a vaginal bladder suspension. They are able to eat on the same day as surgery. Since there is only minimal discomfort, they can be up walking the same day. Walking is the best exercise during the recovery period; it is not too strenuous but gets most of the muscles in the body going again and keeps the circulation moving. However, the sutures still need to heal, and the bladder still needs to form strong scar tissue to hold it in the proper position. Therefore, exercise other than walking and lifting more than 15 pounds still needs to be restricted for three months.

CAN SURGERY BE USED TO TREAT MIXED INCONTINENCE?

In the event that the diagnosis is mixed—both stress and urgency—incontinence, there are several issues to understand before agreeing to surgery. Surgery can put the urethra and bladder back where they belong, but this may cure only the *stress* component of the incontinence. The bladder's errant spasms may continue to cause urge incontinence and wetness. To completely address mixed incontinence, surgery can be combined with any of the other nonsurgical treatments for urge incontinence (see Chapter 5).

Some women with prolapse have both stress and urgency incontinence. Fixing the prolapse will cure both in two thirds of these women. This is especially likely if the urgency incontinence developed only after the prolapse developed. The other third will still require medication to quiet bladder spasms. Women whose incontinence is only somewhat improved by the operation still usually judge the surgery a major success even if they continue to have an occasional spasm or leaking episode.

Katherine's Story

Katherine came into our office seeking a third opinion. She is a forty-six-year-old attorney who spends a good part of her day lugging heavy legal briefs all over town. In addition to a full-time career, Katherine has two children and plays competitive tennis or exercises three times a week. "I'm one of those women who supposedly 'has everything'—career, family, hobbies. But my 'everything' also includes a little bit of burnout and a lot of incontinence," Katherine told us.

Katherine suffered from stress incontinence and was not satisfied with the treatments she had tried so far. Kegel exercises weren't enough, so she was exploring surgical options. One doctor had advised her to have a needle suspension because that was what she did for all her patients with stress incontinence. Another recommended an anterior repair because he'd been doing them for thirty years. He felt comfortable with the procedure and thought it was effective. Katherine hoped there was a solution that really made sense for her particular situation.

In trying to decide which option was best for her, we took into consideration how young, healthy, and active Katherine is. Long-term results were imperative to her. She decided to accept the longer recovery time and increased discomfort that would follow an abdominal bladder suspension because this procedure has the higher long-term success rate.

Katherine was admitted to the hospital and had surgery the same day. The next morning, we went over self-catheterization with her, and her catheter was removed. She started eating regular food and walked up and down the hall that afternoon, just one day after surgery. She did so well that she was able to go home the following day. Within three more days, she was able to urinate with no problems and no longer needed the self-catheterization. Katherine was driving in two weeks and back to work in six weeks. She has continued to do well during the several years since her surgery, with her tennis, exercise, career, and children all intact—a long dry stretch, you might say!

CAN COLLAGEN INJECTIONS BE USED TO TREAT INCONTINENCE?

Now there is a new and effective treatment for one type of incontinence, ISD (see Chapter 1), which has changed the lives of many women who have leaked for years. ISD may be a result of surgery for incontinence that caused excessive scarring or damaged nerves near the urethra. As a result, the urethra does not close properly and leaking occurs. Collagen is a natural substance that adds strength and elasticity to most of the tissues of the body. When taken from cattle and purified for medical use, it has the consistency of thick glue and can be administered by injection. You are probably familiar with the use of collagen by injection since it is commonly used by dermatologists to soften wrinkles in the skin.

The use of collagen for treating incontinence is a simple procedure performed in a doctor's office or hospital, with either local or general anesthesia. A small telescope is placed into the urethra and a small needle is passed through the telescope. The surgeon guides the needle to the portion of the urethra very close to the opening of the bladder. When the collagen is injected into this tissue, it solidifies quickly and causes the urethral lining to bulge inward, making the urethra close off at this point. The partial blockage of the urethra by the bulging collagen helps the urethra stay closed during a cough or upon exercise (Figure 6-4).

This procedure takes only about fifteen to thirty minutes, and the patient goes home the same day. Some women may need to do self-catheterization for a few days until the swelling around the urethra goes down. A few women may note irritation with urination for a day or so, and rarely a bladder infection may occur. No

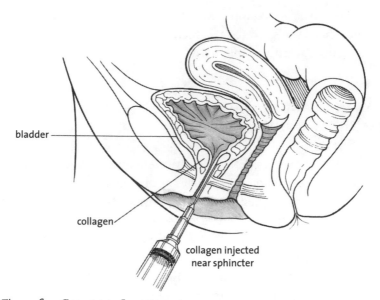

Figure 6-4: COLLAGEN INJECTIONS

long-term side effects have been reported. You can pick up your life where you left off a few days after the procedure. Because about 2 percent of women can have an allergic sensitivity to the collagen, we inject a small amount of collagen into the skin of the forearm a month before the scheduled procedure. If we don't see redness or swelling, we know it is safe to go ahead with the collagen injection procedure.

HOW SUCCESSFUL ARE COLLAGEN INJECTIONS?

Collagen injections bring excellent results, with 80 percent of women having some relief of their symptoms and about 50 percent of women able to stay dry. The success of a collagen injection should be apparent immediately. However, we often find that a series of two or three injections, performed over the course of a few months, is needed to provide these good results. The effectiveness of a series of collagen treatments can last for up to two years. Unfortunately, the collagen dissolves over time, and reinjections usually become necessary. However, if leakage does recur, reinjection can easily be performed. A number of new materials are being developed that are designed to last longer than collagen and therefore might eliminate the need for reinjections.

Although collagen is appropriate for only a small number of women, it is enormously important because it is often successful for women who are the most difficult to cure—namely, those for whom prior surgeries have failed. These women are understandably very grateful for this new technique. Many were our unhappiest patients, but with collagen, they are now dry and satisfied.

Nancy's Story

Nancy is a sixty-three-year-old with her own business that requires some travel. Nancy packs a suitcase for her clothes and a separate tote for her incontinence pads. Fifteen years ago she had a vaginal hysterectomy and anterior repair for mild stress incontinence. She was dry for two years, but then her stress incontinence returned. Three years later, she had a vaginal needle procedure that kept her dry for five years, but then her stress incontinence returned with a vengeance.

She was evaluated again and was told she needed an abdominal bladder suspension, and that excessive scar tissue near her bladder would have to be removed. The surgery was performed, but the leaking returned six months later.

Nancy came to our office at the end of her rope. "How many operations will it take for me to simply be dry? I can't keep doing this." We performed a complete evaluation that showed that the bladder was in the right position but the urethra was open all the time. Nancy had intrinsic sphincter deficiency (ISD). That's why she leaked.

Collagen injections had just become available, and we suggested she try this new technique. A few hours after the injections, she was urinating normally, and she returned to work the next day. She wore her usual large incontinence pad to work (old habits are hard to break) but after three dry days gave them up. The following week, she went on a business trip and packed only her clothes! Over the past three years, Nancy has required two more collagen injections to correct a minor recurrence of leaking, and she continues to be happy and dry.

WHAT IS AN ARTIFICIAL URINARY SPHINCTER?

For women with a severe, otherwise noncorrectable incontinence problem, a surgical procedure can implant an inflatable ring around the urethra. The ring is connected to a small inflating bulb that is placed under the skin to control the opening and closing of the urethral ring. Pressing on one part of the bulb allows the ring to deflate and urine to be passed easily. Pressing on another part of the bulb inflates the ring and keeps the patient dry. This is a difficult procedure to perform but may be indicated for women with an intractable incontinence problem.

WHAT IS INTERSTIM?

Interstim is a surgical method to control symptoms of a hyperactive bladder. Interstim works by electrically stimulating the spinal cord nerves and causing them to relax. Although this is a surgically implanted device, it does not involve surgery on the pelvic organs or muscles. However, since it uses a permanently implanted device, it should be considered only for women who have tried and failed to correct their bladder spasms with other methods. In many people with a hyperactive bladder, the nerves that control the bladder are being activated on their own, without any signals from the brain. As a result, the bladder is almost always in spasm. This unrestrained "noise" occurs between the spinal cord and the bladder in ways that are poorly understood. Your nerves carry impulses in the form of a weak electrical signal. These signals can be interrupted by the stronger electrical signals provided by the Interstim.

The first part of the Interstim procedure is the temporary placement of a small wire near the base of the spine. A temporary device, about the size of a deck of cards, is then used to stimulate the wire to see if the device is effective in decreasing or eliminating the bladder's overactivity. If it is effective, we implant a permanent wire and device.

HOW SUCCESSFUL ARE THESE BLADDER OPERATIONS?

Millions of women are significantly happier because of having had bladder surgery of one type or another. There is an excellent American study that followed women for five years after three different operations performed for stress incontinence. The women who had abdominal bladder suspensions had the best five-year success rate; about 80 percent were still dry. About 45 percent of the women who had vaginal needle bladder suspensions were still dry after five years, and the women with anterior bladder repairs had success rates in the 35 percent range. Sling surgery has a high cure rate, around 90 percent, for women who have previously had a bladder operation that has failed. The procedure has a short recovery period. However, urgency may sometimes follow the operation. TVT is very effective, with success rates around 85 percent after five years.

In addition to success rates, you should consider which procedures are most appropriate for your particular situation. In our own practice we have stopped performing anterior repairs and vaginal needle procedures for the treatment of incontinence because of the low success rates, but it is best to discuss with your doctor which operation is best for you.

HOW CAN YOU DECIDE WHICH OPERATION IS BEST FOR YOU?

Your decision about whether to have surgery at all and, if so, which surgery to have should depend on a number of factors and should be made in collaboration with your surgeon. First, while there may be a number of surgical options for a particular type of incontinence, one operation may be more likely to succeed than others, given your specific test results and symptoms. The severity of the incontinence may also affect your decision. If you have a more bothersome situation, you may be willing to undergo a more involved procedure and a longer recovery to fix the problem.

Other factors that should be considered are your age and general physical condition. The lifestyle you lead is important. If you are not very active and can avoid activities that put stress on your bladder, a less extensive procedure may be enough to correct a problem to your satisfaction. Very active women will often require a more extensive repair to withstand the additional stresses their day-to-day activities put on the bladder.

If you have both prolapse *and* incontinence, the surgery will need to be tailored to fix both problems (see Chapter 10). All these decisions should be made after a careful history and physical examination and proper testing by your doctor. A thorough conversation with your doctor about your problems and wishes should follow. It is also important to ask your doctor which of the procedures he or she is comfortable performing and what kind of success rates he or she has personally had. It may also be a good idea to get a second opinion, preferably from a gynecologist or urogynecologist who performs many of these procedures. All of your needs and concerns should be weighed before you make your final decision.

CAN REPEAT OPERATIONS BE NECESSARY?

While most operations have good long-term success rates, some women may require another operation during their lifetime to correct recurrent incontinence. We know that some of the factors that contribute to incontinence are not yet treatable, such as persistent nerve injury from childbirth or weak supporting tissue due to your own body's innate poor-quality collagen. In some cases, activity may cause sutures to tear out or scar tissue to weaken over time, and the incontinence problem returns. For these reasons, some women may require another operation later in life.

Hannah's Story

Hannah is a nurse assigned to our operating room. We'd worked together for years when she took one of us aside one day and confided that she had a problem with urinary leakage that had gone on for several years. "I'm finally getting up the guts to do something about this," she said.

Her job is very physical, and she found that when she was moving patients or carrying heavy instrument trays, she would leak urine. There was no way to avoid these aspects of operating room nursing, and, as she said to us, "I would be bored taking blood pressures and giving out medications. The operating room is where I really want to be." She saw how many patients we operated on with good surgical results and decided to undergo an evaluation. We knew she loved to travel; she was single without children and did not like the limitations her bladder put on her lifestyle. "Now that I've spoken up about being incontinent, I can't wait to fix it. I wish I'd come to see you sooner."

The examination and evaluation showed a small amount of bladder dropping and a good bladder sphincter, but her urethra moved a lot when we asked her to cough during the exam. With every cough, we could see a small amount of urine leaking.

We discussed the choices and decided to proceed with a laparoscopic bladder suspension, also known as a Burch suspension. She was in the hospital overnight and left the hospital with minimal pain. Hannah was back to most activities within a week. Because her job is so physical, she took six weeks off to recover fully, but we would not allow her to lift anything heavier than 15 pounds for three months and nothing heavier than 25 pounds forever after.

The surgery was successful, and she was happy for years. Unfortunately, after several years of heavy work with the occasional unavoidable need to lift a patient, the problem returned. This time the evaluation and testing revealed that Hannah's urethral sphincter was not closing properly, which allowed the recurrent loss of urine. The remedy for this was collagen injections under local anesthesia until she could take the time to have another surgical procedure. Several months later, during a scheduled leave from work, Hannah had a sling operation as an outpatient. She has since returned to work, dry and pleased, and has arranged with her supervisor that she will never need to lift anything heavier than surgical instruments. She has planned her next vacation and will be leaving for China at the end of the year.

WHAT *LIFELONG* PRECAUTIONS SHOULD BE TAKEN AFTER *ALL* BLADDER SURGERY?

Throughout this chapter, we've tried to emphasize that proper healing and the formation of strong scar tissue take about twelve weeks following surgery. After twelve weeks, major healing has been accomplished, but you will need to continue to protect your bladder repair forever in order to avoid future operations. Therefore, lifting anything heavier than 25 pounds should generally be avoided for life, in order to prevent weakening of the repaired tissue. When you travel, use wheeled luggage or let someone else do the carrying for you. Leave furniture moving to the experts. If you follow these guidelines, your bladder repair is likely to last.

CHAPTER 7

Interstitial Cystitis

With Leslie Kaplan, M.D.

Interstitial cystitis (IC), a bladder condition associated with urgency, frequency, and pelvic discomfort, frustrates those who suffer from it and occasionally even those who treat it. Too often doctors dismiss women afflicted with this uncomfortable disease as being malingerers in need of psychiatric, not medical, care. Too often the women dismissed by these doctors don't realize that they need to see another doctor with another set of diagnostic tools and clinical skills. As a result, they suffer needlessly. Because the symptoms of interstitial cystitis are often confusing and inconsistent, there may be a bit of trial and error before an appropriate treatment begins. If you have been diagnosed with IC or suspect you might have it, we hope this chapter will enhance your understanding of the illness and the available treatments.

If you have a problem with urinary frequency, urgency, and pelvic discomfort and your doctor has not been able to figure out what it is, we hope that reading this chapter will guide you through the maze of medical tests and procedures needed for a diagnosis. Perhaps it will confirm your suspicions that you need a second or third opinion, or simply a doctor with a different area of expertise. Rest assured that you're not alone with this difficult, frustrating problem, and take heart—research on this condition is ongoing.

The medical profession has more to offer IC sufferers now than in the past, but we don't yet have a complete understanding of the problem. You can help yourself by learning all you can to ensure that you get the best possible care. As one of our patients said to us when we told her she had IC, "This disease stinks, and life isn't fair. Now what?" This chapter outlines the best advice we have to offer.

Noreen's Story

Today Noreen, a thirty-one-year-old, seems like a completely different person from the depressed, unhealthy woman who walked into our office three years ago. She talks to us about the feeling of "being in charge of my health again." When we first met Noreen for a consultation, she told us she'd been complaining to doctors about her pain for years. "I couldn't remember feeling really good for at least five years," she said then. She'd been griping to friends, visiting new doctors, trying Chinese herbs, anything to feel better. Her symptoms were cyclical but consistent: pelvic pain that got worse before her period along with urgency and frequency of urination, burning when urinating, and lower back pain. It was quite a load for a thirty-one-year-old to carry. To make matters worse, having sex with her husband had become painful. "Don's a great guy, and I'm afraid he's going to get tired of this soon and want out. I know I'm sick of it. I wouldn't blame him if he leaves me."

She knew she was getting worse, and that scared her. She got up at night to urinate, at first once or twice a night, but then every hour to hour and a half. "I have no strength to fight the pain. I'm exhausted and teary before I even get out of bed. Some days I just don't see how I can keep going."

During the previous five years, Noreen had seen a number of specialists, who had treated her for bladder infections and given her analgesics for the pain, but she didn't feel much better. Two of the doctors had suggested that she seek help from a mental health specialist. She had several friends who were doctors. One suggested that she look for help on the Internet; another sent her to our office.

We began with a history and physical exam. When we did a pelvic exam, we found that her bladder was sore. Her urinalysis and urine culture were clear. We asked her to keep a bladder diary for forty-eight hours, and she documented urinating every one to two hours all night long. We had her come into the hospital for half a day so we could do a cystoscopy under anesthesia. We filled her bladder with 15 ounces of water to see how that affected the bladder walls and saw chronic bladder inflammation. The cystoscopy led us to diagnose moderate to severe interstitial cystitis.

Not surprisingly, Noreen immediately felt relieved when we told her the diagnosis. "I was beginning to believe it was all in my head. Now at least I know I'm not crazy. There's a name for this thing." We assured her that this "thing" was in her bladder, not her head. After discussing all the options, Noreen chose to take an oral medication, Elmiron (pentosan polysulfate), which she would have to take for several months before she felt the positive effects. She also started to instill medications and local anesthesia directly into her bladder, which made her feel better right away. Noreen's Internet search turned up an interstitial cystitis chat room, and we suggested she attend a support group to help her deal with this frustrating condition.

That was three years ago. Noreen still suffers at times, but the pills and the infusions bring relief. The support group ended her isolation, and, to her delight, her husband stuck around. According to Noreen, "He took the 'in sickness and in health' part of our marriage vows seriously, and I love him for it. I'm doing so much better than I was before; even our love life is better. I know what I have; I know what to do about it; and I have a medical team and lots of people behind me."

WHAT IS INTERSTITIAL CYSTITIS?

The truth is, we don't exactly know what interstitial cystitis is. We describe it as a bladder condition associated with bothersome urgency and frequency of urination and/or recurrent discomfort or pain, in both the bladder and the nearby pelvic area. In other words, if you frequently have pain or serious discomfort while urinating and you need to urinate much more often than you used to, you may have IC. For reasons that we don't yet understand, the vast majority of sufferers of IC, upward of 90 percent, are women.

Interstitial cystitis has been known by many other names over the years, including *chronic cystitis, painful bladder syndrome,* and *urgency/frequency syndrome.* A condition often referred to as *urethral syndrome,* originally thought to be a noninfectious irritation of just the urethra, is probably a mild form of IC. Some women who assume they are having recurrent urinary tract infections or think they are getting bladder infections after intercourse may, in fact, have early symptoms of IC. While their urine cultures usually do not grow bacteria, which would indicate infection, these women are often treated with antibiotics all the same. Some women have had persistent symptoms of bladder pain or urinary frequency for months after proper treatment for a true bladder infection. These women may also have IC. The onset of IC is usually gradual, with the symptoms growing worse over time.

So far, despite ongoing research, the exact cause of this condition is not clear. Although this condition was first described in the late 1880s, it was not until the 1970s that the first studies were done to clearly define IC as a condition apart from other bladder problems. And not until 1987 were precise criteria suggested to help doctors reliably establish a diagnosis. It may turn out that IC is an assortment of conditions that all exhibit the same symptoms and therefore seem like the same disease. Or it may turn out to be something we haven't even thought of yet.

WHAT ARE THE SYMPTOMS OF INTERSTITIAL CYSTITIS?

Consistent with the deeply frustrating nature of this disease, interstitial cystitis causes a number of bladder symptoms that can vary from person to person and may even vary in the same individual from time to time. Many women tell us that the symptoms of IC become much worse before their periods. The unpredictability and inconsistency of symptoms make IC difficult to diagnose. That fact has likely contributed to women hearing doctors say, "It's all in your head" instead of the longed-for "Here's what we can do to help." By the time the diagnosis is made, most women with IC have had symptoms for longer than six months, and some for years. That can add up to a lot of suffering and discomfort without even the limited comfort of a diagnosis, let alone treatment.

Most women name bladder discomfort as the most common symptom, and many feel pressure, tenderness, or even intense pain. Women often report the discomfort near the pubic area, where the bladder is located, or near the vagina or the inside of the thighs. Other women experience low back pain as a result of IC.

Most women report that the discomfort is usually worse when their bladder is full. They also feel blessed, but brief, relief after urinating. Because the bladder sits right on top of the vagina, many women with IC have pain with intercourse.

Many women with IC need to urinate frequently (frequency) and often experience a tremendous urge to urinate despite the fact that their bladder is nearly empty (urgency). As a result, while most women urinate six to eight times a day, women with IC pass small amounts of urine approximately sixteen times a day. Needless to say, these women spend a lot of time thinking about and getting to a bathroom. Almost all women with IC need to get up in the middle of the night more than once to go to the bathroom. As the condition gets worse, this need increases. Many women with IC have the sense that they do not fully empty their bladders, even though the bladder is, in fact, empty. Some women find that the urinary stream starts and stops intermittently without much control on their part.

HOW COMMON IS INTERSTITIAL CYSTITIS?

Current figures estimate the number of people in the United States with IC to be as many as 700,000. Ninety percent of people with this condition are women. The average age of women diagnosed with IC is about forty-five, although a few are diagnosed in their late teens. For reasons we don't yet understand, Caucasian women are more likely to have IC than African-American or Asian women, and Jewish women are four times as likely to have IC than non-Jewish women. In addition, women with diabetes appear to be at greater risk.

WHAT CAUSES INTERSTITIAL CYSTITIS?

We really don't know. Scientists and physicians have proposed several theories, but the truth is that we still don't know. Because IC often feels like an acute bacterial bladder infection, one theory suggests that IC may start with such an infection. That theory proposes that an inappropriate immune system response to the initial infection results in the patient's own immune system attacking and injuring the lining of her bladder, leading to the chronic symptoms associated with IC. Other researchers think this is unlikely because bacteria are not found in the urine of women with IC and antibiotics do not resolve the symptoms. A third group feels that IC is an infection that can't be found by common testing because the organism is of an unusual type.

Another theory links IC with the bladder lining cells that produce mucus that coats and protects the cells from the irritating effects of the normally acidic urine. Researchers have identified substances that interfere with the production of this mucus and found that they can produce the symptoms of urgency and frequency just like IC. Yet another theory suggests that an abnormal bladder lining may allow irritating substances to pass into the cells easily and cause the symptoms of IC. Other doctors believe that foods that contain high levels of potassium or are high in acid can cause irritation to the bladder lining in susceptible women. Still others feel that IC may be a condition of the bladder similar to food allergies. While IC has been seen in some mothers and daughters and ethnic groups, a specific genetic link has not been found.

Now you have a sense of why IC is so confusing to both patients and doctors. It may be that there are many causes of what we call IC, but the bottom line is that the bladder responds the same way—with urgency, frequency, and pain—no matter what the cause.

IS INTERSTITIAL CYSTITIS ALL IN YOUR HEAD?

When faced with a confusing set of symptoms, some doctors conclude that the condition must be something psychological. However with IC, this is absolutely not the case. IC is a medical condition of the urinary system.

IC can, however, make women more vulnerable to psychological troubles. As is true with all chronic pain syndromes—low back pain, chronic pelvic pain, temperomandibular joint (jaw) pain—

unrelenting pain that is not easily diagnosed and cured can lead to depression. While antidepressants can alleviate the depression and make the patient feel better, they don't address the cause of the pain. Also, high levels of stress often decrease the brain's tolerance for pain and may make the IC worse. Stress may not cause IC, but stress reduction techniques (see page 169) can often help reduce its symptoms.

HOW CAN THE DOCTOR TELL IF YOU HAVE INTERSTITIAL CYSTITIS?

Unfortunately, there is no test that definitively diagnoses IC. A diagnosis is based on the presence of a combination of symptoms (as described on page 154) without any other definite or obvious cause. Before making the diagnosis of IC, other conditions that can affect the bladder have to be considered and excluded. Those include the following: bladder infection, vaginal or urethral infection, bladder cancer, radiation changes to the bladder, allergic cystitis, bladder stones, endometriosis, ovarian or uterine growths, neurological disorders, and sexually transmitted diseases.

Urethral cultures for unusual organisms and complete vaginal and bladder cultures should be performed. Usually the doctor wants to see you a few times when you are having symptoms and repeat the cultures to make sure they are negative before the diagnosis of IC is even considered. Doctors usually ask their patient to keep a written record, called a bladder diary, of how often they urinate and when pain occurs. This record confirms that urinary frequency is present.

Women suspected of having IC will usually have a cystoscopy under anesthesia (see Chapter 3) as part of their evaluation of bladder symptoms. At that time, the doctor will look for changes in the bladder wall that specifically suggest IC. Hunner's ulcers, damaged areas of the bladder lining, are named for the doctor who first described them. These ulcers were once thought to be hallmarks of IC. However, it turns out that these ulcers are present only in about 2 percent of women with long-standing IC.

At the end of the cystoscopy and while you are still under anesthesia, the doctor can overfill and stretch the bladder with water (hydrodistention). The water is held inside the bladder for a few minutes and let out. In about 80 percent of women with IC the hydrodistention will cause pinpoint bleeding areas on the bladder lining, called glomerulations. This may cause a very small amount of blood in the urine for a few days that then goes away. Glomerulations are not always seen and are sometimes found in women who do not have IC. So this test is not foolproof either.

A biopsy of the bladder lining is sometimes necessary during the cystoscopy, especially if the diagnosis is not clear or, rarely, if there is suspicion of bladder cancer. A pathologist then examines the small sample of lining cells under the microscope. If IC is present, the biopsy may show thinning or even the absence of lining cells, or it may show changes in the cells that typically occur with an immune response. However, a bladder biopsy is not usually needed to diagnose this condition.

Urodynamics testing (see Chapter 3) may also help make the diagnosis of IC. When the bladder is filled with sterile water during the UDS, women with IC usually have a sensation of the bladder filling much sooner than healthy women would. This early sensation of bladder filling is called sensory urgency, a clear sign of IC. While the patient feels this sense of urgency, there are no errant bladder contractions seen during UDS testing. This helps to distinguish women with IC from women with overactive bladders. Another clue found during UDS testing is that the bladder holds only a small amount of water. As mentioned before, women with IC often cannot hold more than 8 ounces in their bladder.

Another test to help diagnose IC is called the *potassium chloride test*. While the patient is awake, a solution of the salt potassium chloride is introduced into the bladder through a catheter. If the bladder lining is covered by healthy lining cells, the patient will not feel anything unusual. However, if the lining cells are abnormal and do not properly protect the bladder from caustic substances, the potassium chloride will irritate the lining cells and cause minor discomfort. The discomfort can quickly be alleviated by placing heparin or Elmiron (pentosan polysulfate) into the bladder (see page 167). Seventy percent of women with IC will have pain during this test.

Joyce's Story

Twenty-five-year-old Joyce knew the uncomfortable feeling too well. This was her third bladder infection, and she decided this time she would see a urologist. "Having a bladder infection is just the worst! I was either in the bathroom or sitting and squirming in pain." Joyce's doctor had prescribed antibiotics, but they didn't seem to help. He switched her prescription to another antibiotic, but still Joyce felt no relief. "Three's the charm, I thought. I tried a third antibiotic, and when that didn't work I told my husband I was ready to say, 'Good-bye, cruel world.' This is intolerable."

Joyce came to our office for a second opinion. We performed a lab test she hadn't yet had. A urethral culture for unusual organisms was positive for a bacteria-like organism called ureaplasm. Although this organism is fairly common as a source of infection, it requires a special culture, so doctors don't often test for it. And the antibiotic required to stop the ureaplasm is different from the ones routinely used for bladder infections. Once Joyce started the proper medicine, the infection cleared up. Within a week she was better. "Good health is such a blessing," she told us. "I'm the happiest woman in town."

WHAT ARE THE CRITERIA FOR DIAGNOSING INTERSTITIAL CYSTITIS?

Since this array of symptoms is crazy-making to everyone—doctor and patient alike—the National Institutes of Health has come up with specific criteria for identifying interstitial cystitis. They are summarized below. These criteria are used primarily for research; by the time a woman meets them, the condition is already far along. As discussed below, the best chance for successful treatment is when the condition is diagnosed early.

A patient must have:
1. Either bladder pain or urinary frequency.
2. Upon examination with the cystoscope, either glomerulations or Hunner's ulcers (see page 157).

A patient cannot *be considered to have interstitial cystitis if she:*
1. Is younger than eighteen years old (IC is not found in younger women).
2. Urinates less than eight times per day while awake or less than two times after bedtime.
3. Does not feel any urgency when her bladder is filled with 5 ounces of water.
4. Has a bladder that can hold more than 12 ounces.
5. Has an overactive bladder as seen during urodynamics (UDS) testing.
6. Has symptoms present for less than nine months.
7. Has symptoms that are relieved by antibiotics or medication for hyperactive bladder.
8. Has another condition that could explain the symptoms, such as a recent urinary tract infection, an active herpes-virus infection, gynecological or bladder cancer in the past five years, or another abnormality of the urethra or bladder.

WHAT CAN BE DONE TO TREAT
INTERSTITIAL CYSTITIS?

Though there are a number of treatments available to treat IC, none of them is universally effective. Bladder training, hydrodistention, dietary changes, medications, pain management, and surgery all have a place in the treatment of women with IC. Each of these treatments is described below. It is best to seek treatment early on because if symptoms have been present for more than a year, the treatments are sometimes less effective. Further research into the causes of and treatments for IC is under way, and we're optimistic that doctors and patients will soon have more treatment tools at their disposal.

CAN BLADDER TRAINING HELP WOMEN
WITH INTERSTITIAL CYSTITIS?

Bladder training can be very helpful for women with IC. Begin by keeping a written record of how often you urinate and how often you feel pain over the next two days (see page 108). You may modify the voiding diary by substituting "pain" for "accidents." Next, calculate the average time between voidings. The following day, add fifteen minutes to the average interval and delay going to the bathroom until that much time has passed since you last made a trip. If you get a strong urge to void, use Kegel contractions or relaxation techniques to delay your next trip to the bathroom until you reach your goal. Each week another fifteen minutes is added to the time between trips until a comfortable schedule is reached. This approach requires patience. It may take a few months to significantly reduce urgency and frequency.

Mary Ann's Story

Mary Ann is a twenty-seven-year-old intensive care nurse at our local hospital. In contrast to the serious illnesses she treated in that unit, she took the discomfort of a urinary tract infection in stride. But the infection was stubborn, and she returned to her doctor several times for treatment. After two courses of antibiotics, the infection finally cleared up. But four months later, Mary Ann still didn't feel well and came to see us for a consultation. "It's not normal to be aware of your bladder all the time. I need to run to the bathroom every few minutes. Something's wrong."

We agreed. The bladder should fill silently, giving us only one or two signals as it fills. Being aware of your bladder all day long is not normal. Diagnostic tests showed that Mary Ann's bladder was still inflamed and irritated by the original infection. The infection was gone, but Mary Ann now had mild interstitial cystitis. We prescribed a course of anti-inflammatory medication and suggested she start bladder training.

Mary Ann took to bladder training with the vigor and determination she devoted to nursing. "I'm going to imagine putting my bladder into boot camp," she told us. "I'm the drill sergeant, and my bladder's the private. This puppy is going to get into shape and behave!" Mary Ann ignored her bladder's demands and stuck to the schedule. In a few weeks, she stopped running to the bathroom all the time. We told her to keep up the training, and within a few months, Mary Ann had only one or two bouts of urgency. By her next annual exam, she told us that she rarely had bladder spasms or urgency. "The case is closed on my misbehaving bladder. I'm very pleased."

WHAT IS HYDRODISTENTION, AND CAN IT HELP INTERSTITIAL CYSTITIS?

Following cystoscopy and overfilling of the bladder (hydrodistention; see page 158) many women will have less pain and a larger bladder capacity. The benefits of hydrodistention can last from four to twelve months. The mechanical stretching of the bladder probably interferes with pain signals transmitted by the bladder nerves and results in a decrease in pain. In addition, the stretching increases the volume of urine the bladder can hold and thus reduces the need to urinate as frequently. About 60 percent of women with IC get relief from hydrodistention.

Janice's Story

Janice is an energetic twenty-three-year-old bank teller. "I'm always closing my window at the bank to run to the bathroom. My manager suggested I switch to a desk position in the loan department, but I really don't want that! The loan department would be so boring. I like being out front where I can talk to the customers and see the sun through the front windows. What's wrong with me?" Janice's frequency, urgency, and even some bladder pain had been causing her problems for six months. The thought of losing the job she liked had finally sent her in search of help. After receiving inconclusive results from all her lab work, we suggested doing a cystoscopy under anesthesia. We saw no pinpoint bleeding, no sores, and no significant scarring, but Janice's bladder was clearly inflamed. We performed a hydrodistention, or overfilling of the bladder with water, in the hope that it would relieve her discomfort.

At a follow-up visit two weeks later, Janice told us she felt much better. "I've been the perfect little teller. I keep my window open until my scheduled breaks, just like I used to do. My manager seems to have forgotten all about the loan department. I hope this lasts for a long time!"

CAN DIETARY CHANGES HELP INTERSTITIAL CYSTITIS?

Some women notice that acidic foods increase the symptoms of IC. A low-acid diet (i.e., avoiding citrus, apples, grapes, tea, tomatoes, and peppers) will often help moderate the symptoms of IC. Also, frequent sips of water will help to dilute irritants and acid in the bladder. However, drinking more than four glasses of water a day may lead to more frequent urination and make the symptoms worse. Calcium citrate, 1,200 to 1,500 milligrams daily, can also help counteract the acidity in your diet. Citrate neutralizes acid in the urine. As an added benefit, the calcium in the pills helps to build your bones. Potassium citrate tablets, 10 milliequivalents three times a day, may also be used to counteract acidity in the bladder.

Stick to a diet of simply prepared rice, potatoes, pasta, vegetables, meat, and chicken. Avoid foods that may irritate your bladder. You'll need to experiment a little to find what foods you can tolerate and which you should avoid. The following foods are known irritants and should be avoided:

Aged cheeses
Sour cream
Yogurt
Chocolate
Onions
Tofu
Soybeans
Tomatoes

Citrus fruits, apples, apricots, avocados, bananas,
cantaloupes, cranberries, grapes, nectarines, peaches,
pineapple, plums, rhubarb, strawberries
Rye and sourdough breads
Smoked meats and fish
Nuts
Alcoholic beverages
Carbonated drinks
Spicy foods
Soy sauce, salad dressings, vinegar

CAN ORAL MEDICATIONS BE USED TO TREAT INTERSTITIAL CYSTITIS?

The medications used to treat IC are administered in two ways: orally (you swallow them) or as solutions placed directly into the bladder (see below). The only oral medication that has shown the effectiveness required to get FDA approval for IC is called Elmiron (pentosan polysulfate). This medication is taken three times a day. How Elmiron helps IC is not clear, but researchers think it repairs the defects in the cells of the bladder that allow the lining to become irritated by the acidity of urine. It takes at least three months before patients experience relief from Elmiron. We recommend sticking with it for six months before giving up on it. If it is effective, patients continue Elmiron for at least one year. Less than 5 percent of women who take the drug will experience side effects, including stomach discomfort and minimal hair loss. Any hair lost during treatment will grow back after the medication is stopped.

Detrol (tolterodine) and Ditropan (oxybutynin) are medications developed to treat frequency and urgency in patients with an overactive bladder, and may help women with IC. Both medications are available as long-acting tablets that need to be taken only once a day. Atarax (hydroxyzine) works well for women who have an increase in pain associated with their menstrual periods. This increased pain is thought to result from an increase in histamine production during that time. Atarax is an antihistamine that can be taken orally to counteract that increase. This medication should also be tried for at least three months. Elavil (amitriptyline) was developed as an antidepressant, but low doses of it and other antidepressants have been found to be helpful for patients with chronic pain of any type. Neurontin was initially used for treating epilepsy, but this drug has also been effective in treating chronic pain syndromes, and it helps some IC patients. L-arginine, an amino acid, and Cytotec, an antiulcer drug, have also been helpful to some IC sufferers. Often doctors combine several of these medications to get a better effect.

Tagamet is an over-the-counter medication developed to prevent excess stomach acid. Prelief is an over-the-counter antacid that can be used prior to a meal to decrease stomach acidity. As discussed on page 164, some women with IC notice an increase in symptoms when they eat acidic foods. These medications help neutralize acids that eventually end up in the bladder.

ARE THERE OTHER MEDICATION OPTIONS?

Yes. Medicated solutions placed into the bladder through a catheter are also used to treat IC. First, the medication is mixed with a sterile solution. A very small catheter is inserted into the bladder and a small syringe filled with the medicine is attached. The syringe pushes the medicine into the bladder and the patient holds the solution there for as long as prescribed. This process is called a bladder instillation. Usually the solution contains a local anesthetic, so the pain relief is often immediate. Most women easily learn to do this at home, and the whole process takes about fifteen minutes.

The only FDA-approved medication for bladder instillation is DMSO (dimethyl sulfoxide), which is effective in about 40 percent of women with IC. Although we don't know exactly how it works, it does reduce bladder inflammation. Instillations need to be done for fifteen minutes weekly for six to eight weeks. The benefits of DMSO can last six months or so. Patients do the instillations at home, and the side effects are minimal. Some patients notice a garlic-like taste in their mouths after the instillation. When tested in animals, long-term use of DMSO has been shown to cause cataracts, although we haven't seen this in people. Anyone using DMSO should see an ophthalmologist every six months for a checkup just to make sure.

Heparin, a commonly used blood thinner, has also been used as a solution for instillation into the bladder. Heparin is similar to Elmiron and may also act to repair the bladder lining. It is effective in about 50 percent of women. Heparin is often combined with a local anesthetic and held in the bladder for about two hours to give relief of bladder pain. Unfortunately, each instillation provides relief from discomfort for no more than a day or so, and instillations need to be repeated five to seven times a week. It may take three to six months of weekly instillations to see any improvement and one to two years before major improvement. BCG (bacillus Calmette-Guérin), a bacterial vaccine used to immunize against tuberculosis, can be mixed with a solution and also used for bladder instillations. It has shown promising results in treating IC.

CAN COMBINATIONS OF MEDICATIONS BE USED?

Many doctors prefer to use a combination of medications to treat IC. We usually start with Elmiron orally and heparin mixed with local anesthetic as a bladder instillation. If bladder pain is a major component of your symptoms, we also give a low dose of an antidepressant. If the pain is cyclical, we may prescribe the antihistamine Atarax by mouth. This combination of medications seems most effective for cyclical symptoms. While the symptoms of urgency and frequency often do not respond to Detrol or Ditropan alone, adding either of these medications to the combination of the other drugs may be helpful. Each combination of medications should be tried for a few months before switching to other combinations. Because every one of us responds to medication in our own unique way, finding the best course of treatment involves some trial and error.

Jodi's Story

Jodi is a forty-five-year-old mother of three sons who gradually developed frequency and urgency over a period of six months. She went in to see her ob/gyn and casually mentioned her symptoms. "I didn't want to make a big thing out of it, but I did tell her my problem. I guess she didn't really listen." During that office visit, her doctor expressed concern about the slight prolapse she detected. She recommended that Jodi have a vaginal hysterectomy and a bladder repair procedure. "I was shocked by the whole thing but figured it was just my time—my mother and my aunts all had hysterectomies. I figured it was my turn."

Jodi went ahead and had the surgery but afterward felt the same urgency and frequency; nothing was different! The ob/gyn assured Jodi that what she was feeling was a normal part of the "healing process" and told her to expect discomfort for at least three more months. Three uncomfortable months passed, and Jodi was no better. She came to our office for a second opinion. We suggested that Jodi have urodynamics testing, but afterward we still weren't sure of the source of the problem. We suggested a cystoscopy and hydrodistention. With her bladder filled with water, we saw the pinpoint bleeding characteristic of IC.

Jodi was shocked. "I never heard of interstitial cystitis, and my old gynecologist never mentioned it. What did I have a hysterectomy for?" We taught Jodi how to do bladder instillations with heparin so she could get relief whenever she felt pain. We also started her on Elavil and Elmiron to minimize her symptoms.

Jodi now tells us she feels much better, and she continues to use the medicines and an occasional instillation to control the IC. "I just wish I'd gone for a second opinion before that hysterectomy. Live and learn."

CAN PAIN MANAGEMENT TECHNIQUES BE USED FOR INTERSTITIAL CYSTITIS?

IC may lead to pelvic muscle spasms that intensify the bladder pain. Thus, learning to relax the pelvic muscles with biofeedback techniques may help. Physical therapy and massage of the affected areas may also help. Your urologist should be able to refer you to a physical therapist knowledgeable about IC. Some women find that exercise, which increases the natural brain relaxants called endorphins, helps relieve some of the discomfort.

Any type of chronic pain can make life stressful and difficult, and a good psychotherapist can provide helpful support. Meditation, self-hypnosis, and stress reduction have all been used to provide relief from the symptoms of IC. Pain management clinics, epidural nerve blocks, or Interstim (see Chapter 6) can be helpful for some women. Since IC often coexists with irritable bowel syndrome (IBS), evaluation and treatment by a gastroenterologist is a good idea if you also have long-standing diarrhea or constipation.

Alternative medicine has been tried with some success by women with IC. Acupuncture has been found to be helpful in 50 percent of women, and herbal therapy may also provide some relief.

ARE THERE SURGICAL TREATMENTS
FOR INTERSTITIAL CYSTITIS?

Despite the fact that there is no known cure for IC, most patients get some relief from medications, distillations, and bladder training. Less than 10 percent of patients ultimately choose surgical treatment. In women who have Hunner's ulcers in the bladder, electricity or a laser can be used during the cystoscopy procedure to destroy the ulcers, leading to significant improvement.

Severe IC can cause the bladder to become scarred and very small. A procedure called bladder augmentation can be performed to add to the storage area for urine. During this procedure the surgeon removes a piece of the patient's intestines and sews it onto the bladder. This increases the size of the bladder. However, because a portion of the bladder itself is left in place, some women may continue to have bladder irritation and continued pain.

Cystectomy, the removal of the entire bladder, is a rare last resort. The surgeon takes a portion of the woman's intestines and makes a pouch inside the body that holds her urine. Obviously, only women who have exhausted all other alternatives and still have chronic pain consider this procedure. Some patients continue to experience pain in the new pouch. The theory is that the same defect of mucus production that is present in the bladder lining probably also exists in the bowel lining cells, leaving them vulnerable to injury from the urine. These women need to continue therapy even after surgery.

Interstim therapy (see Chapter 6) has also been used to relieve the discomfort and urgency of IC. Interstim uses a very mild electric current to interrupt the pain signals going from the bladder to the brain. The first step is the placement of wires through the skin and near the spinal nerves from the bladder. This is attached to an electrical unit worn outside the body. If this is effective, a permanent device, about the size of a deck of cards, is surgically placed under the skin.

ARE NEW TREATMENTS FOR INTERSTITIAL CYSTITIS BEING DEVELOPED?

Due largely to the efforts of patients, IC has become the focus of research efforts by the federal government—the National Institutes of Health (NIH) and the National Institute of Diabetes and Digestive and Kidney Diseases (NIDDK). Drug companies and patient support groups also fund research. Hopefully, as has occurred with breast cancer and prostate cancer research, more attention from patients and doctors will encourage more funding.

Increased funding will be necessary for research to help elucidate the cause or causes of IC and determine which treatments are most effective. Both public education and medical education need to be expanded. We hope that increased awareness on the part of women and their doctors will allow earlier diagnosis and treatment and help prevent the progression of disease to the point where it is difficult to cure.

Efforts are now being focused on how components of the urine or unusual infectious organisms may cause injury to the bladder Hopefully, new treatment strategies will come from these research efforts.

CHAPTER 8

Defining and Diagnosing Prolapse (Pelvic Relaxation)

Sandy's Story

Sandy was twenty-eight years old when her third daughter was born. As a "veteran" of childbirth, she thought she knew what to expect. After this delivery, though, things looked different "down there." She felt a pressure at the opening of her vagina. When looking in a mirror to find out what was going on, she was shocked to see her cervix. "It was as if I was turning inside out," Sandy said. "What used to be inside was just right out there." Sandy told her best friend that it felt like a tampon that was way too low or starting to fall out. Now she often had an awkward, uncomfortable feeling. She felt lucky that she and her husband, Ken, hadn't started having sex since the delivery because she was worried about "how it would work."

In a hurried visit to her obstetrician, Sandy learned she had a uterine prolapse. Since this baby was intended to be her last, the doctor recommended a vaginal hysterectomy. Her obstetrician also told her that sex would be fine even now, especially if Sandy was in a horizontal position. Prolapse is a bit dependent on gravity, and during sex the uterus would slide back to a more normal position. "Gee, you make it sound almost therapeutic," Sandy said. "I wish having sex was the cure. I don't really want an operation."

On the drive home from the obstetrician's office, Sandy began to think that perhaps the doctor's recommendation was hasty and a bit radical. She also fretted about just what this operation would mean to her family. She had a one-month-old nursing infant, a three-year-old in preschool mornings only, and a five-year-old "big girl" who had started sucking her thumb and whining to sit in the infant carrier as soon as the new baby came home. Ken had used up all his vacation days to help out at home after the baby was born. Taking off more days from work without pay would not score any points with his boss and would mean the loss of income they were counting on. There were no grandparents available, either; Sandy's mom lived in Maine and had her own health problems, and Ken's mom had passed away years before.

Sandy's doctor later assured her that the prolapse was not dangerous, and she decided to put up with the annoying sensation until things had settled down a little at home. She said she knew there "just weren't all that many compelling reasons to have a major surgery." After breast-feeding her baby for six months, Sandy realized that the feeling of pressure that had alerted her to the prolapse had gone away. Her cervix was no longer visible unless she really pushed down hard. As far as sex was concerned, Sandy found that everything "worked okay." Time had helped her problem a bit.

She was actually able to ignore the prolapse for years, until her youngest child was ready to graduate from high school. When we saw Sandy in the office, she was forty-six and had recently discovered that her cervix was once again "right out there." Gravity, time, and a midlife change in hormones were causing the uterine prolapse to become a constant annoyance. She came to us for a solution.

After a careful examination, we suggested that Sandy have a vaginal hysterectomy and a bladder repair procedure to fix her prolapse permanently. The postpartum recovery and healing had really helped her prolapse the first time, but we knew she'd need more medical intervention this time. Sandy felt very differently about having a hysterectomy now than when it had first been suggested seventeen years ago. "I know my baby-making days are long over, and I have time to recuperate in peace. I wasn't ready for surgery then, but I have no doubts about it now." Sandy's surgery went well, and she felt very satisfied with the results. "I have no regrets about waiting. My first doctor was a little bit too quick on the trigger for me. The timing now is much better, and it all worked out fine."

WHAT IS PELVIC RELAXATION?

Pelvic relaxation, also called *prolapse,* is the name for the dropping of the uterus or the bulging of the bladder or rectum into the vagina. You can think of it as a hernia, a weakening of tissues that normally hold things in place. Over the past few years, gynecologists and urologists have focused a great deal of attention on the causes of and treatments for weakness in the supporting structures of the pelvis, which leads to prolapse. As the population ages and the number of women with prolapse and incontinence increases, doctors are searching for better ways to help them deal with these problems. And as we develop new methods to help diagnose and treat these conditions, new information will continue to emerge.

For example, magnetic resonance imaging (MRI) has recently been used in research studies to look for changes in the pelvic tissues of women with incontinence or prolapse. Weak muscles and torn connective tissue show up well on MRI, and it is a very accurate way of detecting any damage to the supporting tissues as a result of childbirth, trauma, or aging. The MRI research results show that women with prolapse and incontinence generally have unsuspected damage to areas in the pelvis. We've learned a great deal from these MRI studies, and we are now better able to understand what needs to be done to correct these problems. At this point, MRI is very time-consuming, cumbersome, and expensive and is used primarily for research purposes, but the information from this research will help all women.

Inside the pelvis, a group of muscles shaped like a hammock attaches to the pelvic bones to form a broad area that holds all the abdominal organs in place. When you cough, sneeze, or lift something heavy, the muscles in the pelvis automatically squeeze tight to resist the increase in pressure. Strong connective tissue envelops the uterus, bladder, and rectum and suspends these organs from the bones in the pelvis. When you stand, gravity pulls the intestines and pelvic organs down, but the muscles and connective tissue resist this pull. This well-designed architecture keeps your organs in their proper place (see Figure 1-1).

The vagina and rectum pass through gaps in the middle of the muscle hammock. These gaps create a naturally occurring structural weakness in the muscles. Injuries during childbirth further weaken these muscles and connective tissues, and sometimes result in hernias. Weakening near the bladder allows the bladder to bulge downward; weakening near the rectum allows the rectum to bulge upward; and weakening of the ligaments that support the uterus allows the uterus to slip down into the vagina. These changes are the components of pelvic prolapse.

WHAT DO YOU FEEL IF YOU
HAVE PELVIC RELAXATION?

Oftentimes, especially in mild cases, women will not be aware of any weakening in the areas that support the uterus, bladder, or rectum. For some women, the first sign of prolapse will be a sense of pressure in the vagina. They may even be able to feel a bulge in the vagina with a finger or a bulge coming out of the vagina. This can, understandably, be frightening, and women may associate the bulging with a tumor. But be assured that this bulging is not a dangerous problem; it is *not* cancer and does *not* turn into cancer. If you do feel something, have your doctor examine you so that the type and extent of the problem can be determined. Gravity may pull down on the bladder or rectum and cause pressure or discomfort in the back or pelvis, especially when a woman stands for long periods of time. Lying down often eases the discomfort.

Prolapse is not a serious medical condition, and one of the treatment options, as you will see in Chapter 9, may be to do nothing at all. Some women with prolapse never have any worsening of their condition, while other women have symptoms that become progressively more bothersome over time. Unfortunately, there is no way for the doctor to predict whose condition will worsen. So the choice is really yours. You may choose to seek treatment immediately. But if you don't and the prolapse gets worse over time, treatment is still as close as your doctor's office.

Incontinence sometimes, but not always, accompanies prolapse. In women with severe bulging of the bladder, the urethra can become kinked and the urine flow blocked. In this case, it may be difficult to empty the bladder completely. Difficulty with bowel movements can result from relaxation of the rectum, as the stool may get stuck at the point where there is bulging. Discomfort during intercourse can occur if protruding vaginal skin (which is normally moist and lubricated during sex) becomes dry from exposure to the air.

Elaine's Story

Elaine is in her mid-forties and is the mother of two children. After each birth, she had visible dropping of her uterus and bladder. After her second child was born, her obstetrician recommended a hysterectomy to repair the problem. Since Elaine felt no pain or even discomfort, she dismissed the idea as unnecessary. That was sixteen years ago.

She came to our practice complaining of a "sense of fullness" in the vagina. During the last year, she had felt more and more pressure when she was on her feet or was physically active. "Everything I read tells me to start walking and exercising! But I don't think I can do that with all this pressure. I'm beginning to feel like my life is so restricted." Recently she had seen and felt her cervix at the opening of the vagina, which, in her words, felt "like a tampon that becomes dislodged." When she was lying down, the sensation disappeared completely. Still, she was bothered by the symptoms every day, and she had decided it was time to do something.

Elaine asked, "Have I waited too long to fix this?" We quickly reassured her that if a prolapse is not causing symptoms, it can safely be ignored. There is no medical reason to perform surgery if the prolapse doesn't bother you. However, when it becomes visible and causes pressure, it's time to do something about it.

During the examination, we saw that she had both a cystocele (herniation of the bladder) and a rectocele (herniation of the rectum). We offered Elaine several treatment options, including using a pessary or having surgery. Elaine wanted a permanent solution, so she chose surgery. We suggested removing her uterus through the vagina and repairing both herniations at the same time. Because the symptoms were so bothersome to her, she eagerly agreed. Elaine recovered well from surgery and has no regrets about waiting sixteen years. She told us, "I'm really glad the problem is now fixed, but if I hadn't felt all that pressure, I would never have had the surgery. I'm going to start walking. I feel young again!"

HOW IS THE DIAGNOSIS OF PROLAPSE MADE?

During a pelvic exam, your doctor can look inside the vagina at the position of the bladder and rectum to tell if there is a prolapse. This is done by first taking apart one speculum and placing just the bottom half in the vagina in order to push the rectum down and out of the way, allowing a clear view of the part of the vaginal wall that sits under the bladder. The patient is then asked to cough or bear down. If the areas supporting the bladder are weakened, the bladder will push on the top wall of the vagina and cause a downward bulging (Figures 8-1 and 8-2). The weaker the support of the bladder, the bigger is the vaginal bulge. Bulging of the bladder is called a *cystocele*.

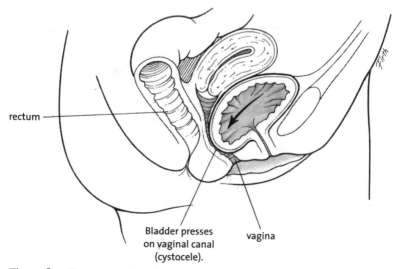

rectum

Bladder presses
on vaginal canal
(cystocele).

vagina

Figure 8-1: CYSTOCELE (SIDE VIEW)

Similarly, by placing the speculum under the bladder, the portion of the vaginal wall over the rectum can be exposed. If the supporting areas of the rectum are weak, coughing or straining pushes the rectum up and the vagina will bulge upward and outward. A bulge of the rectum into the vagina is called a *rectocele* (Figures 8-3 and 8-4). In women who have had a hysterectomy, the small intestine fills the space previously occupied by the uterus (Figure 8-5). If there is a break in the connective tissue at the apex of the vagina, the intestines may push the vaginal wall down. This bulging at the apex of the vagina is called an *enterocele* (Figure 8-6).

In some women, bulging of the vaginal walls occurs only when they stand. Therefore, an examination may need to be performed while you are standing. The doctor can then feel the bulges when you stand and cough. This standing examination might seem a little awkward to you, but it gives your physician needed information.

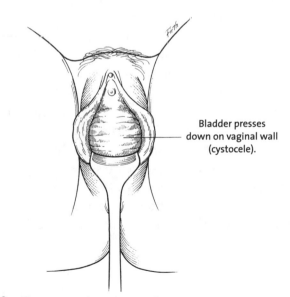

Bladder presses down on vaginal wall (cystocele).

Figure 8-2: Cystocele (front view)

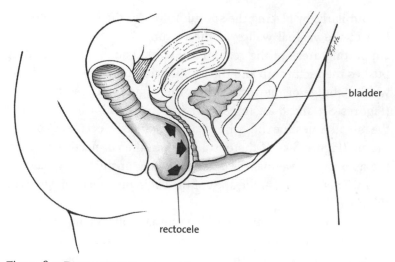

Figure 8-3: RECTOCELE (SIDE VIEW)

WHAT IF YOU HAVE BULGING OF THE BLADDER?

Supporting tissue and muscles suspend the bladder from the pelvic bones and hold it up above the vagina. Childbirth and aging can damage these supporting tissues. As a result of that damage and under the pull of gravity, the bladder may fall down and form a bulge in the vaginal wall called a cystocele. When the bulge is mild, it is usually not bothersome and often goes unnoticed. At the time of a pelvic examination, your doctor may note that you have a mild cystocele, but treatment isn't necessary. If the bulging becomes very pronounced, you may note some pressure inside the vagina, especially after a long day on your feet. If the condition gets even worse, the bulge may be seen or felt at the outside opening of the vagina. If the bulging bothers you, you may want to look into treatment.

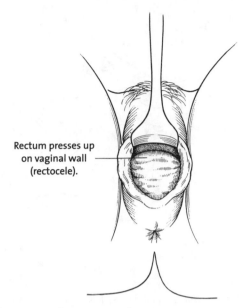

Rectum presses up
on vaginal wall
(rectocele).

Figure 8-4: RECTOCELE (FRONT VIEW)

WHAT IF YOU HAVE BULGING OF THE RECTUM?

Rectal prolapse is the bulging that results from a weakening or tearing of the tissues that hold the rectum down under the vaginal wall. This tissue can be damaged during childbirth and may weaken with age. A rectal bulge is called a rectocele. If the bulge is mild, it often goes unnoticed. More severe bulging can sometimes cause a feeling of pressure in the vagina. In some women, low back pain can occur as the bulging stretches the tissue. Sometimes stool can get stuck in the bulge in the rectum, making it difficult to have a bowel movement. If this condition gets worse, the bulge may be seen or felt near the opening of the vagina. As with a cystocele, a rectocele is not dangerous but can be upsetting and bothersome.

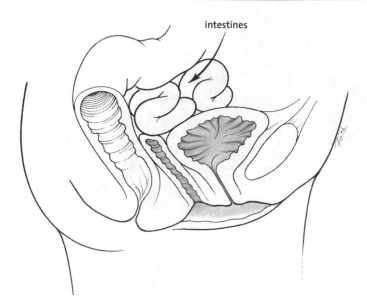

Figure 8-5: NORMAL POSITION OF INTESTINES AFTER HYSTERECTOMY

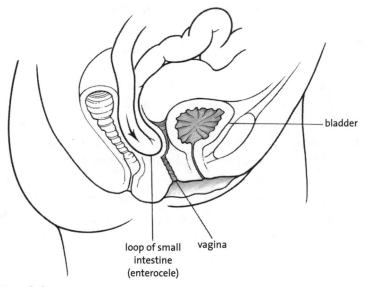

Figure 8-6: ENTEROCELE

WHAT IF THE INTESTINES CAUSE
A BULGING OF THE VAGINA?

Every woman has a small open space in the supporting tissues of the pelvis between the vagina and the rectum. This opening is a naturally weak area, and it does not resist the forces of straining very well. Over time, heavy lifting or straining to have bowel movements may push the intestines down into this area and cause a bulging at the top of the vaginal apex just behind the uterus. This type of bulge is called an *enterocele*. If the uterus has been removed via hysterectomy, the bulging can take up the entire apex of the vagina. Women with this problem may feel pressure in the vaginal area or may have low back pain. As with the other types of weakened areas in the pelvis, this is not a dangerous condition.

WHAT IF THE UTERUS IS DROPPING?

A number of ligaments keep the uterus suspended up inside your torso. The ligaments that do most of this work are called the *cardinal* and *uterosacral ligaments*. These ligaments start just above the cervix and attach to the inside of the pelvic bones. They hold the uterus up and resist the force of gravity pulling it down.

These ligaments are usually stretched during childbirth and weaken further with age. As they weaken, gravity can pull the uterus down into the vagina. This is called *uterine prolapse*. If there is only mild weakening, it is usually not noticeable or bothersome. However, if the uterus drops all the way down to the opening of the vagina, pelvic pressure or even low back pain may result. As with bladder or rectal prolapse, uterine prolapse is not dangerous.

In very rare cases, the entire uterus can drop down and be seen outside the vaginal opening. This is called *total uterine prolapse*

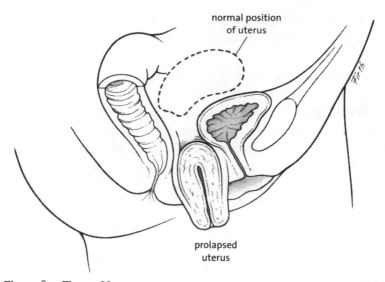

normal position
of uterus

prolapsed
uterus

Figure 8-7: TOTAL UTERINE PROLAPSE

(Figure 8-7). With total prolapse the shift in the position of the uterus can kink the ureters, the tubes that drain urine from the kidneys to the bladder. Total prolapse that kinks the ureters can be harmful to the kidneys, but pushing the uterus back inside the vagina and holding it there with a pessary may solve the problem. Sometimes a pessary does not fit properly or is ineffective, and surgery becomes necessary to correct the problem.

WHAT IS THE POP-Q?

As you might imagine, judging the severity of a bulge is fairly subjective. Many gynecologists use terms such as large, moderate, or small to describe the bulges they see. Others assess the distance the bulge comes down when the patient coughs or strains. For example, if no change in the position of the bladder (or rectum or uterus) is seen, it is called a grade 0. If the bladder comes down halfway to the vaginal opening, it is called a grade 1 cystocele. Grade 2 is bulging to the opening of the vagina, and grade 3 is bulging past the opening. However, this system is subjective and relies on each doctor's estimation of the amount of prolapse.

Recently, a more exact system of measuring these bulges has been developed to try to standardize the evaluation of prolapse for all doctors. This system is called POP-Q, which stands for "Pelvic Organ Prolapse, Quantitative." With this system, the doctor uses a ruler-type device to measure the distance (in centimeters) from the observed bulge to the vaginal opening. If the bulge stays inside the opening, it is expressed as a negative number. As an example, if the bulge is 2 centimeters inside the opening, it would be recorded as −2. If the bulge comes past the opening, the distance is expressed as a positive number. The bulging of the bladder and rectum and the dropping of the cervix are all measured in this way, and the numbers are recorded. This system is very accurate, but it is somewhat more elaborate than previous systems and is being adopted by gynecologists only slowly. At present, all three systems mentioned above are being used to describe prolapse.

Stephanie's Story

"I had to drag her here," said Paula, a longtime patient of ours. "We call her 'Earth mother.' Stephanie takes care of everyone but herself. Need two dozen cupcakes baked? Call Stephanie! Need a place to board your kids and dog for a week? Call Stephanie! I had to threaten her with the disbanding of our car pool if she didn't come in to see you." But Stephanie, a forty-six-year-old mother of four, quickly claimed she'd come in on her own. "I'm so ready to fix all the problems I'm having. Paula gave me a little nudge and offered to buy me lunch afterward. And having a good friend here does give me some comfort and courage."

Stephanie told us she had been thirty-three when she had given birth to her fourth and final child. She'd felt absolutely fine after the birth of number three, but after the fourth, things had been different. "I felt like my organs shifted, and I always felt pressure around my middle." At the time, her obstetrician had told her to wait three months to see if the problems would heal with time. "He was absolutely right," Stephanie said. "I soon felt fine—just like my old self." She eagerly resumed her life, now with a baby always in a carrier, and stayed busy with car pools, assisting the soccer coach, helping set up a Girl Scout troop. "I was thrilled—no feeling of pressure, no symptoms. I thought I'd really dodged a bullet."

Now, thirteen years later, Stephanie's oldest was away at college; her second was getting ready to follow. "Things are quieter at home with just two, and my baby's turning thirteen! I can't believe it!" In the exam room, Stephanie's delight with her children changed to despair about her body. At forty-six, she was having irregular menstrual cycles and occasional hot flashes. During intercourse, her vagina often felt dry and she experienced some discomfort. She complained that by the end of each day, she felt more and more urgency to urinate. "I have no leaking, but, boy, I really feel the need to go all the time," she said. Even a good night's sleep was becoming a sweet memory. Night sweats woke her, and, once awake, she felt an urge to urinate. She then needed to get to the bathroom *fast*. "I worry about making it to the toilet, and once I've gone, I'm so wide awake I have trouble getting back to sleep."

After a complete history and physical, the cause of Stephanie's problems became obvious. She was suffering from a prolapse; her uterus, bladder, and rectum had all dropped considerably. Although she had felt symptoms thirteen years ago, the prolapse had moved back up enough to be undetectable. Now that she was nearing menopause, the old symptoms were back. Four childbirths, hormonal changes affecting the tissues of her pelvis, and the continued pull of gravity had taken their toll. The irregular periods, night sweats, hot flashes, and vaginal dryness could not be blamed on the prolapse, but the urgency and pressure in her abdomen could.

We first had a long talk about hormone replacement and then decided to schedule another appointment so that we could go over the options for repairing the prolapse. "I'm so glad I came in," she said. "And now I'm going to let my good friend Paula buy me that big lunch she promised me."

DO YOU ALWAYS NEED TO BE TREATED FOR PROLAPSE?

Prolapse may cause no symptoms or mild symptoms, in which case treatment is generally not needed. However, some women with prolapse have an uncomfortable feeling of pressure in the pelvis or near the vagina or have back pain related to the prolapse. Some women may be bothered by vaginal irritation or inflammation or may even bleed as a result of the prolapse. For women with bothersome symptoms, some type of treatment makes sense.

The only time treatment needs to be considered for medical reasons is for the rare situation when the uterus falls down to the point that the cervix and most of the uterus can be seen outside the vagina (see Figure 8-6). The uterus, which is partially attached to the bladder, tugs on the bladder and pulls it down as well. If the bladder comes down too far, the ureters may become kinked. If this happens, the urine may not be able to drain from the kidneys and the buildup of pressure may cause kidney damage. Again, this is very, very rare. But if you feel your cervix coming out of your vagina, you should see your doctor for an evaluation.

Except in the case of total prolapse, when your health may be in jeopardy because of kinks in the ureters, it's entirely up to you to decide whether to seek treatment or not. If the prolapse is interfering with your life and your daily comfort, fixing the problem by either surgical or nonsurgical means is worth considering.

CHAPTER 9

Treating Prolapse Without Surgery

Helen's Story

As Helen was known for being blunt, sensible, down-to-earth, and no-nonsense, it came as a great surprise to her family that she had been suffering in silence for years with urgency, incontinence, frequency of urination, and a painful prolapse. "How could I not know?" asked her husband, John. "I knew she went to the ladies' rooms everywhere we went, but I thought all women did that. Boy, I really feel like a clod. I should have known." The truth is that Helen was so masterful at concealing her problem and so convinced that the only solution was a surgical procedure she didn't want that she had told no one—not her friends, not her family, not her doctor. In her words, "Since I'm not willing to have surgery, why bother anyone with this? I just kept it to myself. Plus, who wants to talk about it?" Now sixty-two, she'd been wearing pads for a few years to prevent wetting her clothes. She also had to lie down several times a day to push her cervix back up into her vagina because after she was on her feet for several hours, it would "pooch out."

Helen worked with her husband and son every day in the

family business. Her long-held secret came out when her husband began to plan a lifelong dream—a trip to Europe for the two of them. John told us, "After forty years of breaking our backs to make this business happen, we really deserve a reward. I want to go before we're too old." When Helen knew his plans, she confessed her problem. "I can't be away from home and traveling the way I am," she told him. John insisted she at least ask her doctor what could be done. Helen repeated, "No surgery!" to her internist, who noted the dropping of the uterus and bladder. He referred her to us for specialized care.

When she came to our office, we knew the prolapse needed immediate attention. We fitted Helen for a ring-style pessary. This device looks like a contraceptive diaphragm and fits into the vagina the same way. It took about ten minutes to fit her. The whole process was so easy and painless that it left her speechless. Once the pessary was inserted, it fixed the prolapse entirely. Helen couldn't even feel it inside her. She walked out of the office, pessary in place and absolutely incredulous that relief was so easy.

We asked Helen to come back two days later for a routine check with our nurse practitioner. Fitting a pessary is a bit like fitting shoes. In the store the shoes may feel good, but when you actually start walking in them, there may be a problem. Helen came into the office saying that life was much better but the pessary had fallen out twice. We refitted her with a slightly larger pessary, and she remains deliriously happy to this day. As an added benefit, with the bladder back in its normal position, her urgency, incontinence, and frequency of urination dramatically decreased. Within a month, we received a postcard from Helen and John from Paris.

IF THE SYMPTOMS OF PROLAPSE ARE BOTHERSOME, WHAT TREATMENT IS AVAILABLE?

A device called a *pessary* is a very simple, nonsurgical means of treating a bothersome prolapse. Pessaries were invented more than two thousand years ago. The earliest known pessaries were pomegranates, cut in half and inserted into the vagina to hold the uterus up. Other pessaries were made of balls of wool. A bronze pessary was found in the ruins of Pompeii.

Now pessaries are made of latex and can be placed in the vagina in order to help support the uterus, bladder, and/or rectum (Figures 9-1 and 9-2). Modern pessaries come in many shapes and

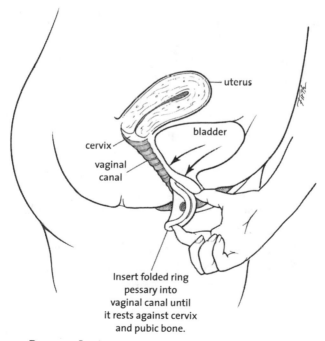

uterus

bladder

cervix

vaginal canal

Insert folded ring
pessary into
vaginal canal until
it rests against cervix
and pubic bone.

Figure 9-1: PESSARY INSERTION

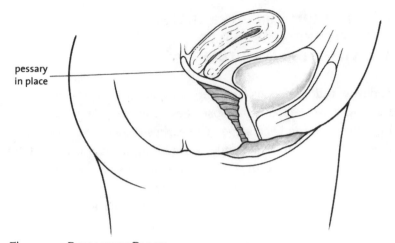

Figure 9-2: PESSARY IN PLACE

sizes, as described on page 193, and many women use a pessary to control troublesome symptoms.

Some women experience symptoms of prolapse or incontinence only during certain activities, such as running, hiking, or exercising. Other women notice a problem only when they are on their feet all day and gravity has time to pull the uterus down. These women may benefit greatly from the use of a pessary. Pessaries are also very useful for women who wish to defer surgery for a while or who are not able to have surgery for medical reasons.

Unfortunately, a pessary does not provide much help for incontinence. It may hold up the bladder well enough to relieve some urinary incontinence. However, in some people, a pessary can temporarily change the position of the bladder in a way that causes the urethra to stay open, and this may increase leaking. If this occurs, you may need to consider surgery.

HOW DOES A PESSARY WORK?

A pessary works by adding a firm support to the weakened tissues inside the vagina. Most types of pessaries use the back of the pubic bone to hold them in place. The top of the pessary pushes the cervix and uterus (or the top of the vagina in women who have had a hysterectomy) back up to a more normal position inside the body. The upper surface of the pessary holds the bladder up, and the lower surface of the pessary holds the rectum down. When fitted properly, the pessary should not move, and you should not be aware that it is in place. The pessary will maintain this support as long as it is in the vagina.

If at times the extra support is not needed, the pessary can be removed. For instance, some women remove the pessary at night, since prolapse is usually not a problem when they are lying down. However, many women leave the pessary in for days, even weeks, at a time. It's easier than removing and reinserting it every day. Pessaries are a temporary solution to prolapse; they work only when they are in place. But many women are able to satisfactorily use a pessary forever and can thus avoid surgery.

WHAT DOES A PESSARY LOOK LIKE?

Pessaries come in many shapes, sizes, and materials. They are often named for their shape or after the person who designed them. Some look like contraceptive diaphragms, others like rubber doughnuts (Figure 9-3). Usually, we can find one that will help. The most commonly used pessary is the *ring* pessary. This looks like a contraceptive diaphragm, except that the middle of the ring is either empty or filled by a thin, flat sheet of silicone. The latex sheet helps to hold the bladder up in women who have a bothersome cystocele. The *Hodge* pessary looks like the ring pessary, except that it is rectangular. This pessary fits under the cervix and

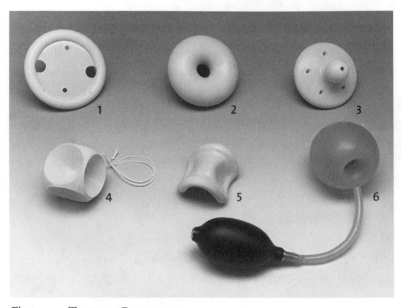

Figure 9-3: TYPES OF PESSARIES

1. RING	2. DOUGHNUT	3. GELLHORN
4. CUBE	5. GEHRUNG	6. INFLATABLE

wedges behind the pubic bone in order to hold the uterus in place. The *Gehrung* pessary is designed to alleviate bulging of the bladder or rectum when the uterus either has been surgically removed or does not need additional support. This pessary is made of pliable plastic and molds itself to fit the contours of the individual. The *Gellhorn* pessary looks like a solid ring pessary with a stem attached to the middle. The stem helps to hold the ring of this stiff pessary in place. The Gellhorn pessary is usually recommended when the prolapse is severe. The *doughnut* pessary looks like a rubber doughnut. One type of doughnut pessary may be inflated to adjust its size as needed, after it is placed in the vagina. Doughnut pessaries are larger than ring pessaries, and we often recommend them if a ring pessary is called for but cannot be fitted properly. A *cube* pessary has six surfaces shaped like suction cups. The suction cups adhere to the vaginal walls and prevent the pessary from falling out. This pessary is difficult to insert and remove, and it needs to be removed frequently in order to avoid vaginal irritation that may lead to vaginal discharge. As a result, we rarely recommend it.

WHERE CAN YOU GET A PESSARY?

Even though pessaries have been around since the time of Hippocrates, many doctors are unfamiliar with their use. Some doctors simply aren't trained to think of them as a way to address prolapse, while others don't think it's worth the trouble to stock a wide range of sizes and shapes in their office. If you are thinking about using a pessary, ask your doctor if the office has pessaries on hand and if he or she is comfortable fitting you for one. If not, you might need to get a second opinion.

A doctor, a nurse practitioner, or a physician's assistant needs to fit the pessary. The process has been compared to fitting shoes. One type of pessary is inserted, and then the patient is given a few minutes by herself to walk around the exam room, bend, twist, squat, cough, and so on to see if the fit is comfortable. She should not be aware of the pessary at all. Several pessaries may have to be tried before the right one is found. The pessary should reduce the prolapse and be comfortable and easy to remove and insert. If the pessary is the proper size, it should be small enough that you are not aware of it at all but large enough so that it does not fall out, even with straining (for example, when you have a bowel movement). And it should not cause incontinence.

A pessary may feel fine in the exam room but start to bother you a few hours later. If the first size is uncomfortable, falls out, or causes leaking, do not be discouraged. Return to your doctor, explain what happened, and another shape or size will be tried. A follow-up visit may be planned within a week of the initial fitting to see if any change is needed. At either the first visit or the follow-up appointment the patient can be taught how to remove and reinsert the pessary herself if she wishes to do so. This is a fairly simple task and can be easily taught in a few minutes.

HOW DO YOU CARE FOR A PESSARY?

If you feel comfortable removing your own pessary, you may do so as often as you like. Some pessaries need to be removed before intercourse. You should wash the pessary with mild soap and water and dry it off with a paper towel. If you remove it for any length of time, store it in a dry place. Pessaries are fairly indestructible and can last for years, though it is not unusual for the latex to become discolored. This discoloration should not cause concern and does not indicate infection or lack of effectiveness. If you notice any cracks in the pessary, however, it should be replaced, since bacteria can grow in the cracks and make infection more likely.

ARE THERE SIDE EFFECTS TO USING A PESSARY?

One possible side effect of wearing a pessary is irritation of the vaginal walls, which can lead to discharge, odor, or, in rare cases, vaginal bleeding. This is not dangerous, but if you have these symptoms, you should see your doctor or nurse practitioner. Estrogen, in either vaginal cream or pill form, may be prescribed to make the vaginal tissues thicker, healthier, and more resistant to irritation and infection. Estrogen also softens the vaginal tissues and makes wearing a pessary more comfortable. If an infection is present, an antibiotic cream will be prescribed until the infection is resolved, and then the pessary can be reinserted. If irritation is chronic or reoccurs, you will probably need to be fitted with a different-sized or -shaped pessary.

In rare instances, the pessary changes the angle of the bladder and urethra and aggravates incontinence. If this is the case, another type of pessary may be helpful. However, sometimes no pessary works effectively, and a woman may need to consider surgery to relieve the symptoms of the prolapse.

WHAT KIND OF FOLLOW-UP CARE IS NEEDED WHEN YOU USE A PESSARY?

If you are able to remove and replace the pessary yourself, some doctors may want you to be examined every few months just to make sure that the pessary is not irritating the vaginal walls. In addition, regular Pap smears and breast and pelvic examinations should be continued as usual.

Some women may not have the manual dexterity necessary to remove and reinsert the pessary. Other women may not feel comfortable placing a device in the vagina. For these individuals, care can be continued at the doctor's office on a routine basis, usually every month or so, depending on how well the pessary fits. Alternatively, if a family member and the patient are both comfortable with it, the family member can be shown how to remove and reinsert the pessary. If you feel any irritation, you should see your doctor. It takes just a few minutes for a doctor to remove it, wash it, and check for irritation of the vaginal walls. If irritation is found at the time of examination, you may have to leave the pessary out for a few days or even weeks, until the vaginal skin heals. If a woman is not caring for herself, her caregiver should be made aware of the pessary and the need for routine follow-up. In rare cases of long-term neglect, a pessary can become trapped or cause severe inflammation or bleeding. If this occurs, the pessary will need to be removed and put aside until the vagina heals fully.

WHEN IS SURGERY NECESSARY?

If using a pessary is not an acceptable option and the symptoms of the prolapse are bothersome, you may choose to have surgery. Remember that treating prolapse is a quality-of-life issue, not a medical one. Except in the rare case of total prolapse, you are not risking your health by choosing to do nothing. However, if your symptoms are very bothersome, you may want to have surgery to put things back where they belong. Surgery should be tailored to your specific problems. If the uterus is falling down and you aren't planning to have additional children, hysterectomy may be warranted. Repair of the bladder and rectum should also be performed, as needed. A full description of surgical options can be found in Chapter 10.

CAN A PESSARY BE HELPFUL BEFORE SURGERY?

Some women choose to use a pessary temporarily until appropriate surgery can be scheduled at a convenient time. Other women may have irritation, inflammation, and even vaginal bleeding due to prolapse. It is best for this to be treated before surgery. A pessary can be used to hold the tissue inside the vagina so that it can heal. Often, an estrogen cream can be inserted inside the vagina nightly to help promote the healing. In addition, the pessary provides relief of symptoms prior to the planned surgery.

Olga's Story

"My Saturday hike keeps me going all week long—without it I think I'd get really depressed," fifty-five-year-old Olga told us. Olga was the sole caretaker of her elderly parents; she did all the shopping, cooking, and cleaning for them, in addition to holding down a full-time job at a local bank. She didn't seem to be getting much help in her own home, either. Her husband "just doesn't see things—like overflowing garbage, dirty dishes, or full laundry baskets." His idea of making dinner was reheating something she'd cooked the night before. "It's just not worth arguing about. I'd rather do it myself," she said.

Her escape from it all is the hikes she takes every Saturday with a local club. But lately she'd felt pressure and bulging in her pelvic area during the hikes and was afraid that she would have to give up this much-needed recreation. She made sure to empty her bladder right before leaving the house, and she tried sucking in her pelvic and stomach muscles. But she still felt a growing discomfort. The rest of the week Olga seemed to be fine. She rarely got that uncomfortable feeling at home or work. "Is there something I can do just for Saturdays?" she asked.

After a physical evaluation, we decided a pessary might be a remedy for Olga's problem. We fitted her with one and asked her to come back for a check to make sure the fit was a good one. Olga's follow-up appointment was on a Monday. She had gone on her hike two days before and came in relieved and happy. She couldn't feel the pessary at all. That Saturday she had been completely comfortable for the first time in a month or two of hikes, and she was delighted.

About two years later Olga came in for her annual Pap smear and checkup. When asked about the hikes and the pessary, Olga was downcast. "It just seems to have stopped working. I have this awful pressure every time I hike. What happened?" It seems that gravity and age had worsened her problem, and the pessary just couldn't do the job any longer. For the most part, Olga was still comfortable except on the hike or after being on her feet for an extended period of time. We tried a pessary of a different shape, but she was still uncomfortable. We started talking about surgery as an option.

"I can take time off work for surgery and recovery, and my

husband can make do without me," she reported, "but I really can't abandon my parents to have this operation. They can't manage on their own at all." On her most recent visit to us, Olga was arranging for her younger sister to come out from Minnesota for a few weeks to care for their parents while Olga had the surgery. In the meantime, she continued to use the pessary while hiking. "It's not the best solution, but I don't want to miss the hike. The pessary will have to do for now."

CHAPTER 10

Treating Prolapse with Surgery

CAN PROLAPSE BE TREATED WITH SURGERY?

While prolapse never leads to serious medical illness, it can make some women's lives uncomfortable or even miserable. As discussed in Chapter 9, some women can effectively treat the symptoms created by pelvic prolapse simply by using a pessary. For some women, though, a pessary is either too difficult or uncomfortable to use or doesn't adequately alleviate the most bothersome symptoms. For those women, surgery can make an enormous difference in the quality of their lives.

Surgical repair of prolapse can be performed through abdominal incisions, through incisions high up inside the vagina, or, more recently, through small incisions in the navel and lower abdomen through which a laparoscope and small instruments are placed. It's common for more than one supporting structure of the pelvis to develop weakness or tears, so it's not uncommon to find that more than one area is in need of repair. The surgical repair of prolapse is undergoing a reevaluation. As noted in Chapter 8, MRI has recently been used to better define the specific areas of damage to muscles and supporting tissues that often lead to prolapse and incontinence. With a better understanding of the problem, doctors have developed new surgical procedures that are more likely to endure over the long run.

Before you proceed with surgery for prolapse, you should understand your particular problem and the treatment options available. This chapter includes an explanation of surgical procedures and the current thinking in urogynecology on each. We hope this information will help when you discuss your situation with a doctor.

WHAT CAN BE DONE IF THE BLADDER IS BULGING?

Repair of a bulging bladder is one of the most common pelvic operations. Weakening or tearing of the supporting connective tissue around the bladder and up inside the vagina can result in bulging of the bladder into the middle portion of the vagina. This weakened or torn connective tissue needs to be surgically mended in order to lift the bladder back to its original position. This surgery involves opening the wall between the vagina and the bladder so that the supporting tissue of the bladder can be seen. The surgeon looks for undamaged connective tissue that can be pulled together and mended. This reinforced tissue holds the bladder in a better position. This procedure is called a *cystocele repair,* and its success rate is excellent.

Sometimes tissue that supports the bladder and connects it to the pelvic bones is torn during childbirth, allowing the bladder to fall down. We call this a *paravaginal defect,* and the result is also a bulging bladder, or cystocele (Figure 10-1). To repair these tears, the surgeon must suture the torn side attachments back together. This repair, called a *paravaginal repair,* pulls the bladder back to its normal position. It may be performed through an incision up inside the vagina, through an incision in the abdomen, or through small incisions in the navel using laparoscopic techniques. Regardless of the type of incision made, the principles of these procedures remain the same; the surgeon's goal is to repair the tissues and return the bladder to as close to its original position as possible.

WHAT CAN BE DONE IF THE RECTUM IS BULGING?

Repair of a bulging rectum is also a common operation. Sometimes childbirth can injure the supporting tissues of the rectum. Weakened or torn tissue will not hold the rectum down in its proper place, and the rectum bulges up inside the vagina. Surgery can repair these weakened or torn connective tissues. The repair is similar in design to a bladder repair. The wall between the vagina and the rectum is opened, and the doctor can actually see and feel the tears just as you can feel a tear in a piece of cloth. Each tear is sutured and closed individually, in a procedure called a *site-specific rec-*

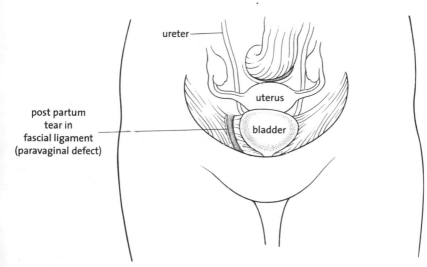

Figure 10-1: PARAVAGINAL TEAR

tocele repair. Once the tears have been fixed, the connecting tissue should be strong enough to keep the rectum in its proper place.

This site-specific repair is an improvement over the previous rectocele repair technique, which depended on thick and inflexible scar tissue forming over the rectum as a result of the surgery. The idea was that this strong scar tissue would reinforce the tissue and hold the rectum down. However, scar tissue in the vagina commonly leads to painful intercourse. One study found that 30 percent of women had stopped having intercourse after a rectocele repair surgery. And once the scar tissue forms, it is almost impossible to remove or fix it. The site-specific repair fixes only the torn parts of the connective tissue and results in much less scar tissue and a decreased chance of painful intercourse. This is a fairly new procedure, so not every doctor is aware of it. The good news is that it is technically easy to learn. If you need repair of rectal bulging, ask your doctor about site-specific repair.

WHAT CAN BE DONE IF THE TOP OF THE VAGINA IS BULGING?

The very flexible small intestine shifts around in the abdominal cavity fairly easily. The cul-de-sac, a small space behind the uterus and directly above the rectum, normally has supporting tissue that holds the intestines up in the abdomen. If this tissue weakens or tears, as can sometimes happen after a hysterectomy, the intestines can drop, creating a bulge in the apex of the vagina (see Figure 8-5). This bulge, called an enterocele, is usually not noticeable to the patient because it is so high up in the vagina. Nor does it usually cause discomfort, incontinence, or other symptoms. However, if other reparative surgery is performed, it is important to fix this problem in order to prevent this weakened area from stretching and weakening other areas of the pelvic supporting tissues. The surgeon performing the hysterectomy can take steps to prevent enterocele formation, but they are limited, and sometimes the tissue weakens despite the surgeon's best efforts.

If an enterocele forms, the idea is to open the apex of the vagina surgically and reinforce the supporting tissues where the intestines push down. This is called an enterocele repair.

WHAT CAN BE DONE IF THE UTERUS IS COMING DOWN?

There are a number of surgical procedures designed to help repair a dropping uterus. As discussed in Chapter 4, the supporting tissues and ligaments of the uterus may undergo an enormous amount of stretching, and even tearing, during childbirth. Together with the changes in the tissues that occur over time, the uterus may drop down into the vagina. This condition is called uterine prolapse.

Many gynecologists feel the best way to treat a falling uterus is to remove it with a hysterectomy and then attach the apex of the vagina to healthy portions of the ligaments up inside the body. Removing the uterus gives the surgeon easy access to the supporting ligaments involved in surgical repair. Some experts also suggest that removing the uterus relieves the strain pulling on the ligaments and increases the likelihood that the repair will last over time. Other gynecologists feel that hysterectomy is a major operation and should be done only if there is a condition of the uterus that requires it. Along those lines, there has been some debate among gynecologists regarding the need for hysterectomy to treat uterine prolapse.

Some gynecologists have expressed the opinion that proper repair of the ligaments is all that is needed to correct uterine prolapse and that the lengthier, more involved, and riskier hysterectomy is not medically necessary. To that end, an operation has been recently developed that uses the laparoscope to repair those supporting ligaments and preserve the uterus. The ligaments, called the *uterosacral ligaments,* are most often damaged in the middle, while the lower and upper portions are usually intact. With this laparoscopic procedure, the surgeon attaches the intact lower portion of the ligaments to the strong upper portion of the ligaments with strong, permanent sutures. This accomplishes the repair without removing the uterus. This procedure requires just a short hospital stay, and recovery is quick. A recent study in Australia found that this operation, called a *laparoscopic suture hysteropexy,* has excellent results. Our practice began performing this new procedure in 2000, and our results have likewise been very good. However, as is the case with all reparative procedures, the goal is the success of the procedure over the long term. Since long-term evaluations are ongoing, ask your doctor his or her opinion about this operation and be sure you understand the reasons for the recommendation.

WHAT CAN BE DONE IF THE ENTIRE UTERUS IS DROPPING?

In rare cases, all of the supporting structures in the pelvis become extremely weakened. As a result, the bladder bulges down, the rectum bulges up, and the uterus drops down and entirely out of the vagina. This is called *total prolapse* or, in medical terminology, *procidentia.* As noted in Chapter 9, a pessary may be used to hold the uterus, bladder, and rectum in place. However, if a pessary does not adequately address your concerns and comfort, it's time to consider surgical options. Because the repairs to each supporting structure need to be made individually, the surgical correction of this problem involves careful attention to each weakened component. In essence, you are having three surgeries, but they are all done at the same time and to the same region and rely on similar techniques.

If you haven't had a hysterectomy, it is usually recommended.

The reasoning here is just a matter of degree; if the ligaments are so damaged as to allow the entire uterus to fall out, repair may not be possible unless the uterus is removed. After the hysterectomy, the bulging of the bladder and the rectal bulge are repaired. In the last step, the apex of the vagina is sutured to the undamaged portions of the supporting ligaments attached to the pelvic bones, moving all the organs back to their normal positions. This surgery, involving careful repair of numerous tissues, takes a few hours.

CAN PROLAPSE OCCUR AFTER A HYSTERECTOMY?

In some women who have had a hysterectomy, the upper portion of the vagina can detach over time from the ligaments that hold it in place. As a result, the top of the vagina can drop down toward the opening. We call this condition *vaginal prolapse.*

There are a number of ways to reattach the top of the vagina to the suspending ligaments on the inside of the pelvis and reestablish the vagina's normal position. These ligaments, called the *uterosacral ligaments,* are often stretched or torn close to the attachments to the cervix. However, stronger, healthy ligaments are usually present higher up in the pelvis. In this area the ligaments are firmly attached to the sacral pelvic bones. One method of suspension uses sutures placed in the ligaments near the sacrum and then pulled through the vagina and tied. As the sutures are tied, the top of the vagina is drawn upward toward the sacrum, back to its normal position. This operation, called *uterosacral vaginal suspension,* is very effective and can be done entirely through the vagina. It requires no abdominal incisions.

Another method of repair sews the apex of the vagina to a strong ligament, called the *sacrospinous ligament.* However, this ligament is off to the side of the pelvis, and as a result the vagina is pulled at a slight angle, usually a little bit down and to the right. This is not noticeable to the patient and does not interfere with intercourse. However, the unusual position can lead to weakening of other support-ing tissues over time. Some surgeons still perform this procedure because this is what they were trained to do. However, most gyne-cologists are now performing the uterosacral suspension because it puts the vagina back into a more natural position.

Miriam's Story

Miriam is an eighty-five-year-old widow who lives alone. She still works part-time in a family gift shop and is quite ac-tive and vital. For many years she'd known she had a uterine prolapse but hadn't been bothered enough by it to pay it much attention. But over the past year, she had felt increased pressure, first occasionally, then daily. Finally, the bulge just wouldn't go back inside her vagina. First we fitted her with a pessary, which helped. However, as the prolapse got worse, the pessary would not stay in, and despite her trying several different types, no pessary took care of the prolapse. She did not want to give up her job and her independence, but the discomfort she experienced while working and shopping for groceries made her life very difficult. She knew she wanted to have surgery, but she was concerned that she was too old.

After undergoing a thorough physical exam, her internist assured her that she could handle surgery quite well. She un-derwent a vaginal hysterectomy, repair of the vagina near the bladder and rectum, needle suspension of the bladder, and suspension of the top of the vagina to the uterosacral ligaments in the pelvis. The day after surgery, she was sore but out of bed and walking. The next day, she was discharged to her home. A visiting nurse checked in on her daily for a week until she was urinating normally, and then we removed her catheter during an office visit. One month later, she was back at her job with no regrets. Spending time on her feet in the store is no longer a painful undertaking, and Miriam is very pleased. She has done extremely well over time and has offered to speak to other older women contemplating surgery to offer them reassurance.

WHAT IS A MESH SUSPENSION?

In some women, the supporting ligaments of the vagina are so weakened or torn that they are beyond repair. For these women, an artificial material can be used to take the place of the weakened ligaments. There are a number of types of materials used to perform this operation, but the most common is a thin, plastic, nonreactive mesh. This mesh is flexible, much like cloth, and can be cut and tailored to fit each woman's anatomy. First the mesh is sutured onto the top of the vagina as it sits inside the body. The vagina is then pulled up to its normal position, and the other end of the mesh is sutured to the connective tissue around the sacral bone to hold the vagina in place (Figure 10-2). The mesh is very strong, and

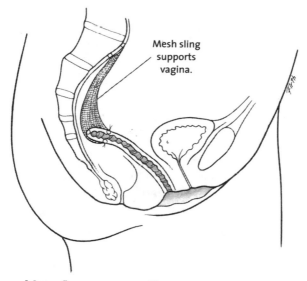

Mesh sling supports vagina.

Figure 10-2: MESH SUSPENSION OF VAGINA

the operation has a high success rate. However, in rare cases, the body can have a reaction to the mesh since it is foreign material. For that reason, the procedure is reserved for women who have had a previous vaginal prolapse surgery that unfortunately didn't do the trick.

This mesh operation is called a *sacral colpopexy* and is most often performed through an abdominal incision. However, recent innovations now allow this procedure to be performed laparoscopically by experienced laparoscopic surgeons. As with other laparoscopic procedures, the hospital stay is shorter and the recovery faster.

CAN LAPAROSCOPIC SURGERY BE USED TO TREAT PROLAPSE?

Laparoscopic surgery requires minimal, $1/2$-inch incisions through the navel and lower abdomen. The benefit of this type of surgery is that patients usually have less pain, a short hospital stay (less than a day), and a return to all but strenuous activity in ten to fourteen days. Laparoscopy was originally developed for the diagnosis of gynecological problems. In the 1970s, some doctors began to experiment with surgical procedures using small instruments specifically designed for the laparoscope. Within a few years, laparoscopic surgeons were performing many operations through the laparoscope. In addition to the benefits to the patient, laparoscopic surgery improves the ability of the surgeon to see into the small spaces of the pelvis. The lighted magnifying telescope actually provides a better view than what the surgeon would see through a larger abdominal incision or with vaginal surgery, in which the narrow spaces in the vagina permit the surgeon an even more limited view.

Today, almost every operation traditionally performed through abdominal or vaginal incisions can be performed laparoscopically, including pelvic repair surgery. The goal of laparoscopic pelvic reconstructive surgery has been to carry over the same principles and techniques used for abdominal surgery. Laparoscopic pelvic reconstructive surgery can thus be used to repair bladder prolapse, uterine prolapse (with or without hysterectomy), vaginal prolapse, and enteroceles. The only area not yet well suited to laparoscopic surgery is the repair of rectal prolapse. However, a site-specific repair of a rectocele can be done after the laparoscopic surgery without difficulty. It should be noted that even though women who have laparoscopic pelvic reconstructive surgery feel well sooner than women who have abdominal or vaginal surgery, it is still important that strenuous activity and heavy lifting be avoided for twelve weeks in order to allow proper healing of the repaired tissues.

When performed by skilled laparoscopic surgeons, the results of reconstructive surgery have been very good. However, since the use of laparoscopy for these operations is fairly new, long-term (five-year) results are just becoming available. The few recently published studies do show excellent results. Laparoscopic pelvic reconstructive surgery requires specialized training and skills. Therefore, if you are considering laparoscopic surgery, you'll want to talk to an experienced gynecologist who performs these procedures regularly.

ARE THERE ANY MINOR SURGICAL PROCEDURES FOR PROLAPSE?

In certain unique situations where a pessary has failed and the patient is elderly, not very healthy, and not physically or sexually active, a minor operation may be used to correct prolapse. This procedure is called the *LaForte procedure*, named after the doctor who developed the operation. First, the prolapsed organs are tucked back inside the vaginal canal. A small amount of skin is removed from the middle sections of the top and bottom of the vagina. The top and bottom of the vaginal walls are then sewn together in the middle, leaving small passageways on either side. These passageways allow mucus or blood from the uterus to pass out of the vagina. When healing occurs, the middle portion of the vagina is closed off, and nothing is able to bulge down into it.

This surgery has many benefits for women who are medically unable to go through more major surgery and who are not sexually active. The operation is relatively simple, has few surgical risks, and can be done as an outpatient procedure with either local, light general, or spinal anesthesia. Recovery is easy, and most women are back to normal activity within a few days. The disadvantage of this operation is that it is not reversible, so the patient should be certain that she does not want to resume sexual activity ever again. Also, closing the vagina may have an effect on a woman's self-image and a sense of femininity. Another possible drawback comes if the uterus is present and abnormal bleeding begins. This usually makes an evaluation with a D and C impossible. As always, every medical procedure has both risks and benefits. Each woman needs to consider all these issues before surgery.

CAN PROLAPSE RECUR AFTER SURGERY?

While our understanding of the changes in the supporting structures of the pelvis is better than ever and our ability to repair these problems with surgery is always improving, there are still areas we do not entirely understand and problems we are not yet able to fix.

For one, we are not yet able to repair damage to the nerves that control the muscles of the pelvis. No matter how well we repair the muscle and other supporting structures, if the nerves can't carry the signals from the brain to the muscles, the muscles won't work properly. Second, some women are born with weak supporting tissue, a condition probably related to the types and amount of collagen these tissues contain. If the tissue is inherently weak, no amount of repair work will prevent it from failing again. Also, as we age, the quantity and quality of collagen decrease and the supporting structures naturally weaken. Therefore, some women who undergo repair of these tissues may have a less-than-satisfactory result or will require surgery again in their lifetime.

Nina's Story

Nina was a thirty-four-year-old mother of two teenage daughters and a nine-year-old son. After her son was born, she had a mild prolapse, which she ignored. Nine years later, her dropped bladder and uterus felt very uncomfortable. "I'll be walking in the supermarket or standing on the sidelines of my daughter's soccer game and just feel this awful strain and pressure. I've started sitting down on the sidelines," she told us. In the last six months, she had also developed mild urinary leakage. "This is all making me so unhappy, but I don't want to have surgery now. I've just got too much going on. Is there anything else I can do?" We fitted Nina with a ring pessary for support, and while she still had minor leaking, she was comfortable and pressure-free.

One year later she decided to have the surgery done over the summer, when her children would be visiting relatives in North Carolina. "My kids will be gone for a month this summer, and that seems like the right time to take care of this," she said. "I'd rather do something fun for that free month, but I'm getting really sick of the leaking. Let's do it in July." Nina had the surgery and was up and active by the time her children came home. The incontinence and the prolapse were successfully corrected.

One afternoon six years later, Nina was horsing around with her now-fifteen-year-old son. "I told him he might be taller than me now, but I'm still stronger. So I proved it by lifting him up. We both laughed, but I immediately knew I'd goofed big time," she said. Lifting more than 25 pounds after a prolapse repair is a mistake. Nina was now back to the same problem she had years before; she had a reoccurrence of the prolapse. To relieve the discomfort she once again felt, we refitted Nina for a pessary, and she is biding her time until she is ready, willing, and able to have surgery again.

CHAPTER 11

Anal Incontinence

With Tracy Childs, M.D.

Bowel movements are a part of our body's function that most of us give no thought to, nor do we care to. However, when problems arise, the effect is profound. As with urinary incontinence, anal incontinence is not life-threatening, but it can lead to restricted activity, embarrassment, social isolation, and depression.

Jessica's Story

Jessica is a young attorney accustomed to living a well-organized, fulfilling life. As with most first-time mothers, her well-organized life went out the window after the birth of her first baby. But that was far from the worst of it. Jessica was passing gas without much control and, on occasion, staining her underwear. During her maternity leave, coworkers in her law firm asked her to come in for lunch to show them the baby. Terrified at the possibility of embarrassing herself, Jessica used the baby's "colic" as an excuse to stay home.

We saw her in our office about six weeks after the baby

was born. The labor had been uneventful, but at the moment of delivery, the baby's heartbeat had gone dangerously low with each contraction. Jessica's obstetrician had felt that a forceps delivery was necessary to protect the health of the baby. The forceps had caused a large tear that went partially through the rectum, and Jessica had needed stitches when it was all over. During her first week home, she could see that some stitches were coming out, and the area seemed greatly inflamed. Soon after, she began to feel as if she was going to soil her pants all the time, and she was having real trouble controlling gas. Her obstetrician assured her that with time the episiotomy and the incontinence problem would heal. About six weeks after the baby's birth, Jessica's episiotomy had healed, but the incontinence problem was, in her words, "really awful." Jessica's obstetrician again told her that more time would correct the problem. She came in to see us for a second opinion. "Just how much time is it going to take for this to go away?"

When we examined her, we saw that the healing had been only "skin deep." The underlying muscles of the area had not healed back together, and her rectum had not closed properly. No matter how much time Jessica gave this problem, it would never heal without surgical repair.

At this point Jessica had another six weeks of maternity leave. She felt ready for an immediate solution and scheduled surgery for that same week. She quickly arranged for child care services and postoperative care and checked in to the hospital. She stayed for four days and pumped breast milk so she could resume nursing her baby as soon as she got home. The surgery, which involved stitching the sphincter muscles of the rectum and anus back together, went very well.

When Jessica came to our office for a six-month follow-up, her smile was as big as baby Sam's. The problem had been completely resolved. Jessica had no worries about the gas or about the need to be near a bathroom. She was back to enjoying motherhood, her job, and her life.

WHAT IS ANAL INCONTINENCE?

Anal incontinence is the uncontrolled passage of stool or gas. Some women stain their underwear or pass gas involuntarily. Others may pass stool without their control or awareness. This is a rare condition in younger women but may be present to some degree in 30 percent of women over sixty-five. The problem is pronounced in more than a third of women with urinary incontinence.

Because it's so painfully embarrassing, few people talk about it. Consequently, no one really knows how common it is. In a large survey of U.S. households, about 1 to 2 percent of the people polled reported a problem with uncontrollable loss of gas or stool. Probably because of childbirth-associated injuries to a woman's rectal sphincter, anal incontinence is ten times more common in females over sixty-five than in males.

Both men and women are more reluctant to talk about anal incontinence than urinary incontinence. One study found that only 5 percent of people with anal incontinence had the problem noted in their medical charts, and another study found that only 30 percent of people with anal incontinence had ever discussed it with their doctors. Clearly, the shame associated with this problem prevents people from getting the help they need. Please understand that anal incontinence is a medical problem, just like an ulcer or diabetes. There are good, effective treatments available. If you have a problem with anal incontinence, we urge you to talk to your doctor.

HOW DOES THE RECTUM NORMALLY WORK?

The stomach, small intestine, and large intestine make up a complex passageway through which our bodies absorb the things we need and eliminate things we don't. The large intestine primarily reabsorbs water into the body. Formed stool remains and is ready for passage. Your body holds this stool in the lower part of the intestine, called the rectum, until you are ready to pass it. The very end of the rectum is called the anal canal. It is the place that sends signals to the brain to help you pass the stool. The anus is the very end of the anal canal and contains the sphincter muscles that hold the stool in. The sphincter muscles are shaped like two tubes, one inside the other. The internal anal sphincter is about one inch inside the anal area, and the external sphincter starts right at the anal opening and extends up into the pelvic floor muscles. The internal sphincter is usually contracted and constantly holds stool in the rectum. The outer, or external, sphincter is normally somewhat contracted, but you can voluntarily contract it further (Figure 11-1).

WHAT ARE THE CAUSES OF ANAL INCONTINENCE?

For women, probably the most common cause of anal incontinence is injury to the muscles and nerves of the pelvis or anus occurring during childbirth (see Chapter 4). Usually the injury is either a tear in the rectal sphincter muscles during delivery or injury to the pelvic nerves from the pressure of either the baby's head or a forceps. There are two pudendal nerves, one on each side of the pelvis, that control the rectal sphincter muscle. Most women will still have good control of the sphincter muscles if just a single pudendal nerve is injured. It appears that injury to both pudendal nerves is what leads to anal incontinence.

There are several other important factors that can lead to anal incontinence. The effect of aging on the tissues and nerves of the

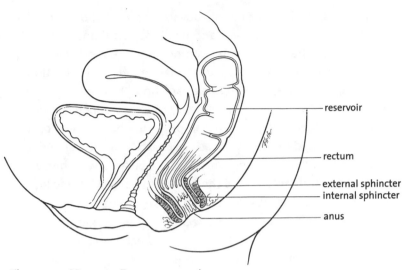

Figure 11-1: NORMAL RECTUM AND ANUS

pelvis can lead to incontinence. Another factor is the individual differences in the types and amount of collagen, which make up the supporting tissues of the pelvis and rectum. Chronic straining when trying to pass stool may, over time, injure the pelvic floor muscles and nerves and make anal incontinence more likely.

One common, and usually correctable, cause of anal incontinence is chronic diarrhea. Often treatment of the diarrhea (see page 222) is all that is needed to solve the problem. Other conditions associated with anal incontinence include diabetes, spinal cord injury, neurological diseases, and injury to the rectal sphincter as a result of previous surgery in that area.

Lauren's Story

Forty-year-old Lauren, a patient new to our practice, approached us with warmth and good humor. She came in because she was leaking small amounts of urine when she coughed or sneezed. This annoyed her, but what really bothered her was incontinence with gas. "I have five children, and my oldest is a fifteen-year-old boy. Pardon my vocabulary, but nothing is funnier to him and his buddies than fart jokes. However, when I pass one, both he and I are mortified. I'm tired of being embarrassed!" Lauren made her situation sound humorous, but she was clearly upset by it.

A year earlier, she'd had surgery to fix a dropped bladder and a bulging rectum. But the problems had persisted. "I originally told my doctor I was okay with the little bulge but upset about the leakage. She was very pleased with herself because surgery corrected the bulge, but I'm still leaking and can't control the gas. Now what?" Our evaluation showed stress incontinence, and we recommended surgery as the best treatment. We sent her to the colorectal surgeon to see if the gas problem could be fixed as well.

The colorectal surgeon evaluated Lauren and found she had an incomplete anal sphincter. Her sphincter had probably torn during one of her deliveries and never healed completely. The surgeon recommended surgery to repair the tear. We performed the surgery on Lauren together, repairing the bladder and the anal sphincter at the same time. Afterward, Lauren's embarrassment was a thing of the past. She can now play tennis and softball with her kids with no worry about gas. "My kids still tell fart jokes, but they're not about me!"

WHAT CAUSES ANAL INCONTINENCE?

The first step in addressing anal incontinence is a discussion with a doctor. This conversation can take place with your family physician, internist, or gynecologist. The doctor will want to know the answers to a number of questions: Are you only passing gas involuntarily, staining your underwear, or actually passing stool without control? When does this happen? Do you have chronic diarrhea? If you have anal incontinence, it is a good idea to have a full evaluation with a colorectal surgeon, a professional trained to take care of these kinds of problems.

A physical exam of the anus can provide evidence of the source of the problem. The doctor will perform a rectal examination and ask you to squeeze the anal muscles. You should be able to close the muscles tightly around the doctor's examining finger. If the muscle does not close tightly, this suggests a problem with either the muscle itself or the nerves that make the muscles function properly. Next, the doctor will touch areas around the anus with a cotton swab to see whether the nerves in this area are working. The doctor will also use the cotton swab to touch close to the anal opening to see if a reflex tightening of the sphincter muscle occurs. A normal reflex shows that the nerves are functioning properly. Most doctors recommend an anoscopy, a test that allows the doctor to look into the anus to see if hemorrhoids are responsible for the staining.

A simple test that can be performed in the bathroom in the doctor's office involves having the patient hold in a small amount of tap water as an enema for about ten minutes. If she is able to do this, adequate anal muscle function is usually present.

IS ADDITIONAL TESTING NECESSARY?

For some women, more involved testing may be necessary to help the colorectal surgeon define the problem. Tests may be necessary to make sure that no other problems, such as inflammatory bowel disease or infection, are associated with the incontinence. Flexible sigmoidoscopy or colonoscopy allows the doctor to inspect the rectum and colon to confirm that everything looks normal.

If the doctor feels the problem may be the result of a previous injury to the anal muscles, usually from childbirth, a test called anal endosonography will usually be performed. This test uses a small ultrasound probe placed into the rectum in order to detect any tears in the rectal muscles. If the muscles are torn, gaps can be seen on the ultrasound monitor.

Another test, called anorectal manometry, measures the pressures within the rectum and anal canal. This test is helpful in determining whether the rectum and anus are functioning properly.

The nerves that go to the pelvic muscles and sphincter muscles can also be evaluated by measuring their electrical activity with small sensors. Surgical repair of the muscles is likely to be successful if there is a gap in the anal sphincter (from childbirth injury) that can be repaired and if the nerves to the muscle are working properly.

Another test that may be performed evaluates the pelvic floor muscles to help determine the cause of the anal incontinence. This test, called videodefecography, is an X-ray test that uses a barium enema in the rectum and colon, plus another liquid material that is swallowed. These liquids can be seen on the X ray. The patient sits on a commode, and a continuous picture is made on the X ray to show how the colon, rectum, and anus function during straining and passing stool.

ARE THERE MEDICATIONS THAT HELP TREAT ANAL INCONTINENCE?

One frequently treatable cause of staining or loss of stool is chronic diarrhea. It is certainly harder for the anal sphincter to hold fluids than to hold solid stool, and staining or leaking stool may result. The doctor may perform a colonoscopy to make sure that you do not have any obvious causes of diarrhea, such as an infection (infectious colitis) or inflammatory bowel disease (ulcerative colitis). A stool sample will be tested for parasites. If no cause of the diarrhea is found, medications can be given to help control the loose stool. Over-the-counter medications called *bulking agents,* such as

Metamucil or Citrucel (methylcellulose), are most commonly used to help firm the stool. There are also medications such as loperamide (Imodium) or, by prescription, diphenoxylate with atropin (Lomotil) that slow down the action of the intestines, allowing the large intestine to absorb more water from the stool, making it firmer.

Some women have anal incontinence because they have had damage to the pelvic nerves and have a diminished sensation of stool in the rectum. They cannot anticipate when they need to go to the bathroom. These women can regularly use an enema to help keep the rectum empty so that no accidents occur. A simple tap-water enema can be used after a bowel movement to clean out any remaining material. Enemas may also be used if other medications have not been successful.

Meredith's Story

Meredith, a tall, trim accountant in her early sixties, decided to "really start paying attention to my health." She purchased only organic produce and began a regimen of dietary supplements—lots of vitamins and herbal potions from the health-food store. "I really had no compelling reason to start taking all those things, but it just seemed like a good idea. Turning sixty kind of shook me up."

Meredith didn't feel much different once she began all the supplements, and taking them just became part of her daily routine. Within a few months, she began to suffer from diarrhea. "I thought I had some kind of stomach bug at first." But the diarrhea didn't stop, and Meredith found herself soiling her underwear, especially as she neared the bathroom. She tried eating lots of rice and cutting down on fruits and vegetables, but the diarrhea persisted. And now the soiling happened much more frequently.

When she mentioned the problem to her family doctor, he inquired whether there had been any changes in her diet or whether she was taking any medications. She casually mentioned the herbal supplements and extra vitamins, and her doctor suggested she stop taking them to see if that made a difference. The next step would be to check her for intestinal parasites and anal sphincter problems, but the doctor felt suspicious about the supplements. Meredith cut back and started taking only calcium and a multivitamin every day. Within three weeks, the diarrhea and anal incontinence were gone. "What a relief! To think I was trying to keep myself healthy with all that stuff."

CAN PELVIC MUSCLE TRAINING WITH BIOFEEDBACK HELP WOMEN WITH ANAL INCONTINENCE?

Biofeedback employs the same principles in treating rectal incontinence as it does in treating urinary incontinence. The goal is to retrain the muscles in order to regain control. Basically, the training teaches women to be more aware of the sensation of stretching of the lower colon as it fills with stool. By becoming aware of this feeling and then contracting the pelvic floor, they can learn to hold their stool in. Biofeedback training uses the same equipment that is used for teaching pelvic floor exercises. However, to retrain the sphincter muscles, a small balloon is placed just inside the anus and slowly filled with air. Another catheter is placed higher up in the rectum. When the woman feels the air filling the rectum, she is asked to voluntarily contract the rectal sphincter for ten seconds. Once the monitor shows that the patient is contracting the proper muscles, the patient is instructed to contract the muscles for ten seconds three times a day.

The goal of biofeedback is to teach the patient to keep the anal sphincter contracted while relaxing the pelvic muscles. The patient can see how well the sphincter contracts on a monitor. Biofeedback works fairly well in women who have a problem with control after anal or rectal surgery. If the sphincter has been injured or torn as a result of childbirth, the muscle will not function properly despite these exercises.

Biofeedback is often successful. In fact, about 70 percent of women will have some improvement. Some progress is seen immediately after biofeedback, and the improvement may be sustained for several years after treatment.

ARE THERE SURGICAL TREATMENTS FOR ANAL INCONTINENCE?

Women who have tears of the rectal muscles from vaginal childbirth are the most likely to benefit from surgery. Repair of the muscles involves opening the skin over the muscles, finding the ends of the torn muscles, and sewing them in an overlapping pattern to give added strength. While complete continence is difficult to achieve, significant improvement often results in 70 to 90 percent of women.

More complicated surgical repairs have been developed for women who do not have enough working, healthy muscle left to put back together. One such repair uses the gracilus (thigh) muscle. A small portion of the thigh muscle is cut and brought down to the rectum to reinforce the area. This surgery can be helpful for about 60 percent of people with this problem.

ARE NEW TREATMENTS FOR ANAL INCONTINENCE BEING DEVELOPED?

In most areas of surgical medicine, research is proceeding to develop artificial body parts to replace our own parts that no longer work properly. In colorectal surgery there is very active research for an artificial anal sphincter that can be surgically implanted around the anus. A balloon in the artificial sphincter can be filled when the patient wants to hold stool in and deflated when the patient wants stool to pass. Recently, collagen injections, similar to those used in the urethra for urinary incontinence, have successfully solved the problem of anal incontinence. A topical gel that contains a medication called phenylephrine has been used to cause the sphincter muscle to contract. Patients can apply the gel before they need to go out, and the effect will last for several hours.

CHAPTER 12

Sexuality

Our sex lives are sometimes hard for us to talk about. We struggle to tell our children "the facts of life," and we struggle to tell our partners what pleases us. Sex is personal and, at its best, is an intimate treasure, savored privately. We all want to please and be pleased, to feel warm, safe, and desired. For many women, perceived problems with their weight, overall appearance, and desirability can cause enormous anxiety. When a woman chooses to have sex, oftentimes her worries and insecurities get right into bed with her. Does he like my body? Am I pretty? Are my thighs too big? As you age, those issues may make you more ill at ease. Add prolapse or incontinence to the mix, and things can get pretty complicated. Incontinence may turn that small, still voice of insecurity into a loud roar.

Shelley's Story

Forty-two-year-old Shelley has been a patient in our practice for fifteen years. We were there at her children's deliveries and got updates on her son and daughter at each of Shelley's annual checkups. Since our own families and children were around the same ages, we shared stories about school, soccer, and Scouts. She once said, "I know I can talk to you about anything." But one day in the office she admitted that despite feeling that closeness, she still hadn't been able to mention one "terrible problem."

"I've tried to bring this up every time I have a physical, but it is just so embarrassing. Even my husband and I don't discuss it. This mortifies me to tell you, but I leak urine every time I have an orgasm! I know you gave me lots of opportunities to bring this up, but I just couldn't get past my own embarrassment."

We were very glad she finally told us because we have many remedies for her problem. We decided to start with the easiest solution—biofeedback and pelvic muscle exercises. Shelley began the exercise program that afternoon and progressed rapidly. In four months, her leakage was under control. As an added bonus, pelvic floor strengthening increased her sensitivity during intercourse, and her stronger vaginal muscles added to her husband's experience too. "Boy, am I happy I finally found the courage to tell you. I might have missed out on so much."

DOES INCONTINENCE AFFECT YOUR SEXUALITY?

The good news is that a recent study tells us women with incontinence or prolapse report having the same amount of sexual activity, comfort, and enjoyment with sex as women without incontinence. There's more: 80 percent of the women with either prolapse or incontinence felt their partners were also satisfied with their sexual relationship. Naturally, a woman's feeling about her partner and the relationship has a lot to do with whether she is satisfied sexually or otherwise. But the incontinence and prolapse turn out to be less important than expected. Incontinent or not, many women stay sexually active well into their seventies and eighties.

However, the same study stated that women with the most severe prolapse or most frequent incontinence did report that their physical condition interfered with their sex lives. As a result, these women were more distressed about their medical situations and were less content. While the women with less severe incontinence did not have a significant problem with sexual satisfaction, those with severe problems found they were detrimental to their sex lives.

CAN YOUNG WOMEN HAVE INCONTINENCE DURING SEX?

Surprisingly, young women actually have incontinence during intercourse more than older women. A study performed in Israel found that while only 3 percent of women over age sixty-five reported incontinence with sexual activity, 29 percent of women under age sixty had this problem. And, as might be expected, this incontinence caused these women some anxiety. While almost all the women in this study were in stable marriages, 43 percent of them felt anxiety because of the incontinence during intercourse. Although there is no comparable study for single women, more than likely the absence of a stable relationship only makes things worse.

CAN INCONTINENCE CAUSE A PROBLEM WITH SEX?

Incontinence makes some women feel unclean and consequently undesirable. They may consequently avoid sex or feel less pleasure and freedom when they do have sex. The type of incontinence a woman has can greatly affect how much it troubles her. Women with stress incontinence usually have fewer problems with sex than women with urgency incontinence. Stress incontinence often happens at predictable times, most often right at the beginning of intercourse, when penetration alters the angle of the bladder and urethra. Urinating just before having sex usually prevents this problem. Urgency incontinence, the result of an overactive bladder, causes more distress because it is unpredictable and unavoidable. Women with urgency incontinence often lose urine during an orgasm, which may be particularly upsetting. Also, the amount of urine leaked because of an overactive bladder is usually greater than with stress incontinence. One study found that almost 70 percent of women with urgency or urgency incontinence had unsatisfying sexual relations, while only 20 percent of women with stress incontinence had this complaint.

Leslie's Story

Leslie is a forty-three-year-old computer programmer who has two grown children and is now eagerly awaiting her second marriage. When she came in for a checkup, she was exasperated. "How can I possibly have a romantic wedding night when I've got this cervix at the opening of my vagina?" She told us that little by little her cervix had been descending and was actually visible when she stood for long periods of time or was very active. "I'm too embarrassed to even discuss this with my fiancé, and the wedding is next month. What can I do?"

During the physical exam, we determined that Leslie had a uterine prolapse. After a long discussion, Leslie understood that when she was having intercourse, the cervix and uterus would just move back in, and her fiancé would not feel or notice anything amiss. We suggested she use a diaphragm for contraception, which would also help keep her uterus in place during intercourse.

When Leslie came in six months later for her annual exam, she glowed with good health and happiness. "Everything is wonderful—I feel like I'm on a perpetual honeymoon." That was five years ago, and her cervix, diaphragm, and marriage are all holding strong.

CAN PROLAPSE CAUSE PROBLEMS DURING SEX?

Prolapse does not usually cause problems during sex. If prolapse results in bulging of the bladder or rectum into the vagina, the bulge can easily be pushed back into place before intercourse, and most women with prolapse say they don't notice it during intercourse. Also, if you have a prolapse, you should know that intercourse will not cause any harm to whatever is bulging: your bladder, vagina, uterus, or rectum.

It is common for women to notice that the prolapse is much less apparent when they are lying down, a likely position during sex, which allows the prolapse to move out of the way. However, if the prolapse is severe, the vagina may be exposed to the drying effect of the air and intercourse may be irritating and uncomfortable. In that situation, a lubricant can be very helpful.

Mary's Story
"They say your first love is really your true love, and I am about to find out if there's any truth to that," said Mary, a seventy-eight-year-old widow. Her first love, Howard, a man she had not heard from in forty years, had come back into her life out of the blue. Mary's brother, who lived in a distant city, had received a call from Howard, asking for Mary's address. Howard had recently lost his wife to cancer and had a yearn-

ing to see if Mary was alive, well, and available. He'd needed to do a fair amount of scouting around to come up with Mary's brother's phone number. According to Mary, he felt as though he'd "won the lottery" now that they were back in touch.

Mary had been incontinent for seven years when she came to our office. She had never wanted surgery and was basically comfortable wearing pads. But now she and Howard planned to reunite, and Mary did not want to greet a lost love or even think about a romantic weekend wearing incontinence pads.

We suggested she try the FemAssist for a few days to see if it would work for her. The FemAssist is a small adhesive-backed plastic patch that can be placed over the urethra to prevent leaking. Within a day, she knew she'd found the solution she needed for the reunion weekend. As long as she had the patch on, she had complete protection. She was able to remove the patch whenever she wished and was able to avoid surgery.

"The weekend was a dream come true for me, and so was finding such a simple solution for such an awful problem," she said. Mary and Howard spent a lot of time catching up on forty years of living. They found comfort and companionship with each other. "We are very special friends, and I'm not so lonely anymore. That patch really helped me start a new phase in my life. I am just thrilled."

DOES INCONTINENCE MAKE YOU LESS ATTRACTIVE?

Incontinence can undeniably complicate life in an unpleasant way. Many women modify what they wear and how they live as a result. Some tell us they feel less feminine and less independent. They limit their wardrobe to dark clothing in order to hide any possible leaks. They avoid situations where they won't have easy access to a bathroom. Some women so dread embarrassing themselves that they feel comfortable only at home. They may also be concerned about odor and may fear that nobody will want to sit next to them at social events. However, as we hope readers will learn from this book, there are now many ways to prevent incontinence. The social and physical isolation that incontinence sometimes brings is unnecessary.

HOW CAN YOU TALK WITH YOUR PARTNER ABOUT INCONTINENCE?

Both women and men with incontinence may suffer from feelings of isolation. Embarrassment and fear of humiliation often keep them from talking to their partners about the subject. Usually the fear is worse than the reality. Unnecessary tension and emotional distancing hurts both people in the relationship. We know that good communication between lovers helps to make sex more joyful under any circumstance. If you have incontinence, talking to your partner about it may be the most important thing you can do. Good communication will lead to greater affection and trust. Talking about any kind of problem is usually easier in a long-term, intimate relationship, but even in a new relationship, getting things out in the open often brings relief.

If you have incontinence during intercourse, discussing this with your partner before having sex might help you both. Many women, although embarrassed at first, are surprised at how easily the conversation goes. Oftentimes mentioning that there might be a bit of dribbling is all that is needed. Some men worry about getting a bladder infection from an incontinent partner. Although loss of urine may feel unclean, urine is entirely sterile. You can reassure your partner that there is no risk of transmitting infection. Others worry needlessly about hurting a woman with a prolapse when all that is needed is to push the prolapse back and use a lubricant. The bottom line is very clear: incontinence does not need to get in the way of sexuality.

SHOULD YOU DISCUSS SEXUAL PROBLEMS WITH YOUR DOCTOR?

If many women have problems talking to their partners about sex, isn't it even more difficult for them to broach the subject with their doctors? To complicate things even further, doctors are often uncomfortable about discussing sex and are rarely well trained to do so. Adding incontinence to a conversation may make both a woman and her doctor even more reluctant to pursue further discussion.

To illustrate what a significant problem this is, interviews with 324 sexually active women found that only 2 women had volunteered information about having incontinence during sex. However, when specifically asked about this symptom, 77 additional women acknowledged that they had had incontinence during intercourse.

Patients and doctors need to do a better job communicating about incontinence and sexuality. If your doctor doesn't ask about incontinence, it is important for you to bring it up if there is a problem. If your doctor seems uncomfortable with the subject, ask for a referral to someone who regularly deals with incontinence. If you are having a problem with incontinence and sexuality, more than likely you will need to bring this up as well. If your doctor is not equipped to discuss it with you, ask for the name of a knowledgeable therapist who can help. If your doctor doesn't know such a specialist, make an effort to find someone on your own (see Chapter 13). The important thing is to get what you need. You're not alone with this problem.

CAN KEGEL EXERCISES PREVENT
LEAKING DURING SEX?

Kegel exercises can certainly help. Women who learn to do Kegels correctly and do them regularly (see Chapter 5) have less leaking during intercourse. A recent study from Norway found that women who were taught the correct way of performing Kegels by a physical therapist were more likely to have more satisfying sex than a group of women who were not properly taught these exercises. The women had fewer problems with their sex life and less discomfort during intercourse. We encourage you to do Kegel exercises on a regular basis.

WHAT ELSE CAN HELP PREVENT
LEAKING DURING SEX?

Another way to prevent leaking during sex is to keep your bladder reasonably empty during intercourse. Try to avoid drinking fluids for an hour or so before you expect to have intercourse. This will keep the bladder from filling up too quickly once you get into bed. If you empty your bladder just before you begin lovemaking, leaking is much less likely.

WHAT ARE THE BEST POSITIONS
TO PREVENT LEAKING?

Some positions make leaking much less likely. A woman on top has control over penetration and better control of her pelvic muscles. Some women find more control in positions they find less tiring. Intercourse on your side is usually less strenuous. Rear entry will keep pressure directed away from the bladder and urethra.

However, everyone is different, so you should experiment with different positions until you find the ones that work for you.

WILL SEX BE BETTER IF YOU HAVE SURGERY?

To answer this, a recent American study questioned a group of women before and after surgery to repair a prolapse or incontinence. About half of these women were sexually active. Before surgery, 82 percent of the sexually active women reported being happy with their sex lives, and after surgery, 89 percent of the women felt happy with their sexual relationship.

The study brought out a number of interesting findings. First, the frequency of intercourse did not change following surgery. Second, while only 8 percent of the women had pain during intercourse before surgery, 19 percent noted pain during intercourse after surgery. About one quarter of the women who had had a repair of a bulging rectum (rectocele) developed pain during intercourse. About one third of the women who had had repair of a rectocele and a bladder suspension had painful intercourse. Unfortunately, the researchers did not ask these women why they were more satisfied with their sex lives even though more of them had painful intercourse.

Another study performed in Sweden may shed some light on this mystery. This study found that one third of women noted an increased interest in sex after incontinence surgery, and one half of their male partners were more interested in sex. It could be that knowing that the prolapse or incontinence had been surgically addressed was enough to make the couples feel better about sex.

WHAT CAN YOU DO IF INTERCOURSE IS PAINFUL?

One way to reduce discomfort during intercourse is to use a lubricant. Ask the pharmacist to recommend a good lubricant, or try a few to see which one works well for you. Avoid Vaseline or hand lotion, as these tend to dry out quickly. If vaginal dryness is a long-standing problem, consider asking your doctor about vaginal estrogen. Estrogen makes the vagina more elastic and increases natural lubrication. Local forms of estrogen, available as creams, estrogen-containing silastic rings, or small pills inserted into the vagina, can improve vaginal health without any significant absorption of the estrogen into the bloodstream and the body.

IF YOU HAVE INTERSTITIAL CYSTITIS, CAN ANYTHING HELP MAKE SEX MORE COMFORTABLE?

For a woman with IC, finding out what works for her and her partner can involve some trial and error. In general, women tell us that sexual positions where the pressure is off the bladder are the most comfortable. Many report that the most comfortable position is lying on their side or rear entry. Again, the best idea is to experiment until you find what works for you. Some couples substitute oral sex if intercourse is too painful. Using a vibrator to stimulate only the clitoris without involving the vagina may also give pleasure. Putting a heating pad on the pelvic area before sex brings blood to the area and may help facilitate orgasm. A cold pack applied on the pelvic area after sex helps keep inflammation and discomfort down.

HELPFUL HINTS TO A BETTER SEX LIFE

Here are bits of information that our patients with incontinence have told us helped them improve their sex lives:

1. This is the most important and obvious: Be sure you have an understanding partner. Talk to your partner about your situation. Whether you are incontinent or not, a supportive, caring lover is what you need. Make sure you have the partner you deserve or help your partner become one. Seek professional counseling if necessary.
2. Always empty your bladder before intercourse. This should help you avoid leaks and maximize your enjoyment.
3. Try to avoid fluids just before intercourse. This doesn't mean you need to be dehydrated or dry-mouthed, but avoiding that cup of coffee or cola may make a big difference.
4. If you think you might need them, use towels, disposable pads, or rubberized sheets to keep the bed dry and fresh. Planning ahead may minimize any anxiety you have.
5. Be calm if you leak. Urine is a sterile fluid, and a little leakage is just not that important. A sense of humor might help defuse the situation, while anger or frustration may only increase your anxiety or that of your partner. Sometimes our bodies seem to be loaded with booby traps for potential embarrassment. That's the way we humans are.
6. Do Kegel exercises regularly. Well-toned muscles often decrease or eliminate leaking, and they can increase pleasure for both partners.
7. Experiment with your partner to find the most comfortable positions for you both.

CHAPTER 13

Finding the Right Doctor

By our best estimate, there are about 15 million women with incontinence or prolapse in the United States. If each one of them sought medical care for this problem, the thirty thousand gynecologists practicing today would not have enough time to evaluate and care for them all. And most gynecologists (and urologists) have not been properly trained to care for these women. It was only about twenty years ago that several gynecologists and urologists began focusing on helping women with incontinence and prolapse and created a subspecialty field called urogynecology. As a result of the efforts of these doctors, there has been great progress in the evaluation and treatment of these problems. With new developments, and with the likely increase in the number of women having incontinence and prolapse as the baby-boom generation ages, the number of doctors trained to treat incontinence and prolapse will likely also increase. In recognition of this growing need, the American Board of Obstetrics and Gynecology and the American Board of Urology have joined forces to accredit a new subspecialty fellowship called Female Pelvic Medicine and Reconstructive Surgery. Three years of fellowship training in women's incontinence and prolapse will be necessary for certification. As of 2002, about fifteen hospitals have accredited training programs in this new specialty, with more to be added each year. The establishment of this new fellowship validates the concept that urogynecology is now a priority for women's health care.

We hope that the topic of women's incontinence and prolapse will enter the public's awareness and that women will begin to discuss these conditions instead of suffering in silence. We hope that word will spread to women that there are good medical solutions to incontinence and prolapse. It is important to find a doctor who has the training and experience necessary to provide you with the best care currently available.

ARE ALL PRIMARY-CARE DOCTORS TRAINED TO TREAT INCONTINENCE?

Unfortunately, the answer is no. Most family doctors or internists receive very little training about women's incontinence. And since many women and their doctors find incontinence a difficult subject to discuss, patients and doctors avoid initiating discussions. This is the main reason that the National Institutes of Health felt it necessary to publish federal practice guidelines for all U.S. physicians instructing them about the evaluation and treatment of incontinence. If you have a problem with incontinence, we urge you to bring it up with your doctor. If you are in a managed care plan, you may need to ask for a referral to a gynecologist, urologist, or urogynecologist in order to receive the proper care.

ARE ALL GYNECOLOGISTS TRAINED TO TREAT INCONTINENCE?

Most gynecologists have received some training in women's incontinence and prolapse during their residency. However, residency programs vary with regard to the expertise of the teaching faculty, and some programs spend very little time training the residents to evaluate and treat incontinence properly. Therefore, the amount of training and the level of interest of gynecologists vary greatly. Obstetrician/gynecologists, especially those recently trained, spend a fair amount of time doing obstetrics and primary care for women. While women thus enjoy access to a doctor they know well who provides a broad range of primary care, obstetrical, and gynecological services, this gives the doctor less time to learn and maintain specialized surgical skills.

For these reasons, if you have incontinence or prolapse, it is probably best to find a doctor who has a special interest in these areas and who has taken the time to get extra training. If a physician is actively engaged in treating the complex problems of incontinence and prolapse, he or she will likely read urogynecology subspecialty medical journals and newsletter updates about current therapy and research, and attend urogynecology conferences. Most gynecologists with an interest in female incontinence belong to the American Urogynecologic Society (AUGS). It is important that you try to find a doctor who has the special training and expertise in incontinence and prolapse.

Recently the fields of urogynecology and laparoscopy have intersected. Much pelvic reconstructive surgery can now be accomplished with laparoscopic techniques performed by experienced laparoscopic surgeons. Many of the gynecologists with interest and expertise in laparoscopic surgery belong to the American Association of Gynecologic Laparoscopists (AAGL). If you think you have a problem that may be amenable to laparoscopic surgical repair, consider finding a physician who has interest and expertise in both areas. Looking through the member lists of AUGS and AAGL may help start that search.

ARE ALL UROLOGISTS TRAINED TO TREAT INCONTINENCE IN WOMEN?

In general, most urologists spend the majority of their time dealing with male urological problems such as prostate trouble because they are more common than female incontinence. Urologists with no particular interest in female incontinence are often inadequately prepared to treat prolapse and incontinence comprehensively. Vaginal surgery, bladder repairs, hysterectomies, and rectal repairs are not routinely included in urology surgical training programs. Those surgical techniques belong to the gynecologist. However, some urology residency programs do teach these skills, so if you are being treated by a urologist, ask if he or she can provide comprehensive care.

WHAT IS A UROGYNECOLOGIST?

Since most gynecologists have incomplete training in care for women with incontinence and prolapse, a new subspecialty was formed to focus on female urology and pelvic surgery. Because the field combines urology (specializing in the bladder, kidneys, etc.) and gynecology (specializing in the female reproductive system), the new field is called urogynecology. A urogynecologist is a doctor who completes the full training in gynecology and then gets further training in the evaluation and treatment of female incontinence and pelvic prolapse.

In addition, many gynecologists and urologists have an interest in the problems of female incontinence and prolapse. These doctors spend considerable time learning about those problems and gaining the needed expertise for the proper evaluation and treatment of bladder and prolapse problems. Additionally, a gynecologist and a urologist may team up to work together or consult with each other for difficult problems. A colorectal surgeon is consulted when there are problems with anal incontinence. This multidisciplinary approach works extremely well.

The American Urogynecologic Society, in conjunction with the American Urological Association, promotes the education of gynecologists and urologists in the treatment of women with incontinence and prolapse. AUGS, as it is also called, has about seven hundred members who have shown such an interest. If you contact the American Urogynecologic Society, it can give you names of members in your area. Some university medical centers have departments of urogynecology whose staff members teach and see patients. Your family doctor or internist may also be able to recommend a physician with special expertise in this field.

HOW SHOULD YOU CHOOSE A DOCTOR FOR YOUR BLADDER OR PROLAPSE PROBLEMS?

Experience counts, and in medicine it counts a great deal. This is where you need to be your own advocate by asking lots of questions. Here are some questions we think are worth asking the doctor:

1. Do you often treat women with incontinence or prolapse?
2. How much extra training in treating female incontinence and prolapse have you received?
3. Do you work as part of a team with other gynecologists, urologists, and colorectal surgeons?
4. What other tests are available to evaluate my specific condition?
5. Do you regularly offer urodynamics (UDS) testing?
6. What are the alternatives to the treatment you are recommending for me?
7. How many of these surgeries have you done? What is your success rate?

8. Are you recommending this surgery because it is what you usually do? Is it the best choice for my particular needs? Do you perform it several times a month?
9. Is laparoscopic surgery reasonable for the condition that I have?
10. Are you trained in laparoscopic procedures, and do you perform them frequently?

We suggest you read the parts of this book that relate to your particular situation carefully. Write down any questions you may have and take them with you when you visit your doctor again. Look for a gynecologist, a urogynecologist, or a gynecologist and urologist working together in order to find a satisfactory solution to your problem. Ask if both your urologist and gynecologist have experience treating your particular problem.

SHOULD YOU GET A SECOND OPINION?

We think getting a second opinion is an excellent idea, especially if surgery has been recommended. Very few things in medicine are black or white, and there are often differences of opinion. Don't worry about hurting your doctor's feelings. The vast majority of physicians are very comfortable about their patients' seeking another consultation. Most of them would likely do the same thing for themselves or their family members. If you are facing surgery, you will have peace of mind if you've done all your homework and have sought the best care possible.

When patients in our practice get a second opinion, we ask them to call and talk to us about the results of that consultation. This allows us to answer any new questions and respond to any suggestions the other physician has offered. If we disagree with the recommendations, we can also explain why. We never feel offended if a patient wants a second opinion. Remember, this is your body and your health. Do not be afraid to get another opinion.

WHO SHOULD YOU CONSULT
FOR A SECOND OPINION?

Seeking a second opinion sometimes seems awkward. Here's how we recommend you go about doing it.

First, tell your gynecologist that you want another opinion. Just be up front and tell him or her you want another professional's thoughts about your case. Your doctor will likely appreciate your honesty and may be able to provide you with the name of a gynecologist, urologist, or urogynecologist who is well respected. Another alternative is for you to call a nearby university-based medical center to see if it has a urogynecology department. Also, your family doctor or internist may know gynecologists or urologists in the community who are knowledgeable about urogynecology.

If you find a physician for a second opinion without your own doctor's help, consider notifying your doctor of the name of this second physician. That will give him or her an opportunity to voice any concerns about the recommendations you have been given. This need not dissuade you from seeking care from another doctor, but you will at least be aware of any differences of opinion.

HOW CAN YOU BE SURE OF GETTING GOOD CARE?

In this book, our aim is to educate you about problems with incontinence and prolapse and to present state-of-the-art information regarding a range of solutions. We want to help foster a healthy doctor-patient partnership, something we believe is vital to good care. It is in your best interest to be educated about the health care decisions you make. If you need more information, seek it out. Get a second opinion. Ask all the questions you need until you understand and are comfortable with the answers. Seek out information about possible alternatives. When it comes time to make decisions, you will feel confident and secure about your choice.

Chapter 1: Defining Incontinence

Blaivas, J. "The Neurophysiology of Micturition: A Clinical Study of 550 Patients." *Journal of Urology* 127 (1982): 958.

Diokno, A. "Diagnostic Categories of Incontinence and the Role of Urodynamic Testing." *Journal of the American Geriatric Society* 38 (1990): 300.

Elving, L., A. Foldspang, G. Lam, and S. Mommsen. "Descriptive Epidemiology of Urinary Incontinence in 3,100 Women Age 30–59." *Scandinavian Journal of Urology and Nephrology* 125 (suppl.) (1989): 37.

Herzog, A., and N. Fultz. "Prevalence and Incidence of Urinary Incontinence in Community-Dwelling Populations." *Journal of the American Geriatric Society* 38 (1990): 273.

Kelleher, C., L. Cardozo, and P. Toozs-Hobson. "Quality of Life and Urinary Incontinence." *Current Opinion in Obstetrics and Gynecology* 7 (1995): 404.

Klutke, C., J. Golomb, Z. Babaric, et al. "The Anatomy of Stress Incontinence: Magnetic Resonance Imaging of the Female Bladder Neck and Urethra." *Journal of Urology* 143 (1990): 563.

Nygaard, I., F. Thompson, S. Svengalis, et al. "Urinary Incontinence in Elite Nulliparous Athletes." *Obstetrics and Gynecology* 84 (1994): 183.

Chapter 2: How the Bladder Normally Works

McGuire, E. "The Innervation and Function of the Lower Urinary Tract." *Journal of Neurosurgery* 65 (1986): 278.

Walters, M. "Mechanisms of Continence and Voiding, with International Continence Society Classification of Dysfunction." *Obstetrics and Gynecology Clinics of North America* 16 (1989): 773.

Chapter 3: Diagnosing Incontinence

Byrne, D., P. Stewart, and B. Gray. "The Role of Urodynamics in Female Urinary Stress Incontinence." (1987)

Jensen, J., F. Nielsen, and D. Ostergard. "The Role of Patient History in the Diagnosis of Urinary Incontinence." *Obstetrics and Gynecology* 83 (1994): 904.

Karram, M., and N. Bhatia. "The Q-tip Test: Standardization of the Technique and Its Interpretation in Women with Urinary Incontinence." *Obstetrics and Gynecology* 71 (1988): 807.

Scotti, R., and D. Meyers. "A Comparison of the Cough Stress Test and Single-Channel Cystometry with Multichannel Urodynamic Evaluation in Genuine Stress Incontinence." *Obstetrics and Gynecology* 81 (1994): 430.

Versi, E., G. Orrego, E. Hardy, et al. "Evaluation of the Home Pad Test in the Investigation of Female Urinary Incontinence." *British Journal of Obstetrics and Gynecology* 103 (1996): 162.

Wyman, J., S. Choi, S. Harkins, et al. "The Urinary Diary in Evaluation of Incontinent Women: A Test-Retest Analysis." *Obstetrics and Gynecology* 71 (1988): 812.

Chapter 4: Childbirth and Incontinence

Allen, R., G. Hosker, A. Smith, and D. Warrell. "Pelvic Floor Damage and Childbirth: A Neurophysiologic Study." *British Journal of Obstetrics and Gynecology* 97 (1990): 770.

Chiaffarino, F., L. Chatenoud, and M. Dindelli, et al. "Reproductive Factors, Family History, Occupation and Risk of Urogenital Prolapse." *European Journal of Obstetrics and Gynecology and Reproductive Biology* 82 (1999): 63.

Connolly, A., and J. Thorp. "Childbirth-Related Perineal Trauma: Clinical Significance and Prevention." *Clinical Obstetrics and Gynecology* 42 (1999): 42.

Handa, V., T. Harris, and D. Ostergard. "Protecting the Pelvic Floor: Obstetric Management to Prevent Incontinence and Pelvic Organ Prolapse." *Obstetrics and Gynecology* 88 (1996): 470.

Meyer, S., P. Hohlfeld, C. Achtari, and P. De Grandi. "Pelvic Floor Education After Vaginal Delivery." *Obstetrics and Gynecology* 97 (2001): 673.

Meyer, S., P. Hohlfeld, C. Achtari, et al. "Birth Trauma: Short and Long Term Effects of Forceps Delivery Compared with Spontaneous Delivery on Various Pelvic Floor Parameters." *British Journal of Obstetrics and Gynaecology* 107 (2000): 1360.

Norton, P. "Pelvic Floor Disorders: The Role of Fascia and Ligaments." *Clinical Obstetrics and Gynecology* 36 (1993): 926.

Snooks, S., M. Swash, S. Mathers, and M. Henry. "Effect of Vaginal Delivery on the Pelvic Floor: A 5-Year Follow-up." *British Journal of Surgery* 77 (1990): 1358.

Sultan, A., and S. Stanton. "Preserving the Pelvic Floor and Perineum During Childbirth—Elective Cesarean Section?" *British Journal of Obstetrics and Gynaecology* 103 (1996): 731.

Chapter 5: Treating Incontinence Without Surgery

Arya, L., D. Myers, and N. Jackson. "Dietary Caffeine Intake and the Risk for Detrusor Instability: A Case-Control Study." *Obstetrics and Gynecology* 96 (2000): 85.

Boyington, A., and M. Dougherty. "Pelvic Muscle Exercise Effect on Pelvic Muscle Performance in Women." *International Urogynecology Journal* 11 (2000): 212.

Brubaker, L., T. Harris, D. Gleason, et al. "The External Urethral Barrier for Stress Incontinence: A Multicenter Trial of Safety and Efficacy." *Obstetrics and Gynecology* 93 (1999): 932.

Burgio, K. "Behavioral Training for Stress and Urge Incontinence in the Community." *Gerontology* 36 (suppl.) (1990): 27.

Miller, J., D. Perucchini, L. Carchidi, et al. "Pelvic Floor Muscle Contraction During a Cough and Decreased Vesical Neck Mobility." *Obstetrics and Gynecology* 97 (2001): 255.

Miller, K., D. Richardson, W. Siegel, et al. "Pelvic Floor Electrical Stimulation for Genuine Stress Incontinence: Who Will Benefit and When?" *International Urogynecology Journal* 9 (1998): 265.

Von Kerrebroeck, P., K. Kreder, U. Jonas, et al. "Tolterodine Once-Daily: Superior Efficacy and Tolerability in the Treatment of the Overactive Bladder." *Urology* 57 (2001): 414.

Chapter 6: Treating Incontinence with Surgery

Das, A., M. White, and P. Longhurst. "Sacral Nerve Stimulation for the Management of Voiding Dysfunction." *Reviews in Urology* 1 (2000): 43.

Liu, C. "Laparoscopic Treatment of Genuine Stress Incontinence." *Clinical Obstetrics and Gynecology* 8 (1994): 789.

McGuire, E., and R. Appell. "Transurethral Collagen Injections for Urinary Incontinence." *Urology* 43 (1994): 413.

Meltomaa, S., A. Haarala, M. Taalikka, et al. "Outcome of Burch Retropubic Urethropexy and the Effect of Concomitant Abdominal Hysterectomy: A Prospective Long-Term Follow-up Study." *International Urogynecology Journal* 12 (2001): 3.

Scotti, R., A. Angell, R. Flora, et al. "Antecedent History as a Predictor of Surgical Care of Urgency Symptoms in Mixed Incontinence." *Obstetrics and Gynecology* 91 (1998): 51.

Ulmsten, U., C. Falconer, P. Johnson, et al. "A Multicenter Study of Tension-Free Vaginal Tape (TVT) for Surgical Treatment of Stress Urinary Incontinence." *International Urogynecology Journal* 9 (1998): 210.

Chapter 7: Interstitial Cystitis

Gillenwater, J., and A. Wein. "Summary of the National Institute of Arthritis, Diabetes, Digestive and Kidney Diseases Workshop on Interstitial Cystitis, National Institutes of Health, Bethesda, Maryland, August 28–29, 1987." *Journal of Urology* 140 (1998): 203.

Parsons, C. "Interstitial Cystitis: Clinical Manifestations and Diagnostic Criteria in over 200 Cases." *Neurourology and Urodynamics* 9 (1990): 241.

Parsons, C., G. Benson, S. Childs, et al. "A Quantitatively Controlled Method to Prospectively Study Interstitial Cystitis and Demonstrate the Efficacy of Pentosanpolysulfate." *Journal of Urology* 150 (1993): 845.

Parsons, C., and P. Koprowski. "Interstitial Cystitis: Successful Management by a Pattern of Increasing Urinary Voiding Interval." *Urology* 37 (1991): 207.

Wein, A., and G. Broderick. "Interstitial Cystitis: Current and Future

Approaches to Diagnosis and Treatment." *Urology Clinics of North America* 21 (1994): 153.

Chapter 8: Defining and Diagnosing Prolapse (Pelvic Relaxation)

Aronson, M., S. Bates, and A. Jacoby. "Periurethral and Paravaginal Anatomy: An Endovaginal Magnetic Resonance Imaging Study." *American Journal of Obstetrics and Gynecology* 173 (1995): 1702.

Bump, R., A. Mattiasson, K. Bo, et al. "The Standardization of Terminology of Female Pelvic Organ Prolapse and Pelvic Floor Dysfunction." *American Journal of Obstetrics and Gynecology* 175 (1996): 10.

Norton, P., C. Boyd, and S. Deak. "Collagen Synthesis in Women with Genital Prolapse or Stress Urinary Incontinence." *Neurourology and Urodynamics* 11 (suppl.) (1992): 300.

Schull, B. "Pelvic Organ Prolapse: Anterior, Superior, and Posterior Vaginal Segment Defects." *American Journal of Obstetrics and Gynecology* 181 (1999): 6.

Chapter 9: Treating Prolapse Without Surgery

Emge, L., and R. Durfee. "Pelvic Organ Prolapse, Four Thousand Years of Treatment." *Clinical Obstetrics and Gynecology* 9 (1996): 997.

Sulak, P., T. Kuehl, and B. Shull. "Vaginal Pessaries and Their Use in Pelvic Relaxation." *Journal of Reproductive Medicine* 38 (1993): 919.

Chapter 10: Treating Prolapse with Surgery

Benson, J., V. Lucente, and E. McClellan. "Vaginal Versus Abdominal Reconstructive Surgery for the Treatment of Pelvic Support Defects: A Prospective Randomized Study with Long-Term Outcome Evaluation." *American Journal of Obstetrics and Gynecology* 175 (1996): 1418.

Iosif, C. "Abdominal Sacral Colpopexy with Use of Synthetic Mesh." *Acta Obstetricia et Gynecologica Scandinavica* 72 (1993): 214.

Lyons, T., and W. Winer. "Minimally Invasive Treatment of Urinary Stress Incontinence and Laparoscopically Directed Repair of Pelvic Floor Defects." *Clinical Obstetrics and Gynecology* 38 (1995): 380.

Maher, C., M. Carey, and C. Murray. "Laparoscopic Suture Hysteropexy for Uterine Prolapse." *Obstetrics and Gynecology* 97 (2001): 1010.

Ross, J. "Apical Vault Repair, the Cornerstone of Pelvic Floor Reconstruction." *International Urogynecology Journal* 8 (1997): 146.

Ross, J. "Laparoscopic Burch Repair Compared to Laparotomy Burch for Cure of Urinary Stress Incontinence." *International Urogynecology Journal* 6 (1995): 323.

Shull, B., S. Benn, and T. Kuehl. "Surgical Management of Prolapse of the Anterior Vaginal Segment: An Analysis of Support Defects, Operative Morbidity, and Anatomic Outcome." *American Journal of Obstetrics and Gynecology* 171 (1994): 1429.

Ulmsten, U., C. Falconer, P. Johnson, et al. "A Multicenter Study of Tension-Free Vaginal Tape (TVT) for Surgical Treatment of Stress Urinary Incontinence." *International Urogynecology Journal* 9 (1998): 210.

Vancaillie, T. "Laparoscopic Colposuspension and Pelvic Floor Repair." *Current Opinion in Obstetrics and Gynecology* 9 (1997): 6.

Webb, M., M. Aronson, L. Ferguson, et al. "Posthysterectomy Vaginal Vault Prolapse: Primary Repair in 693 Patients." *Obstetrics and Gynecology* 92 (1998): 281.

Weber, A., and M. Walters. "Anterior Vaginal Prolapse: Review of Anatomy and Techniques of Surgical Repair." *Obstetrics and Gynecology* 89 (1997): 311.

Chapter 11: Anal Incontinence

Den, K., D. Kumar, J. Williams, et al. "The Prevalence of Anal Sphincter Defects in Faecal Incontinence: A Prospective Endosonic Study." *Gut* 34 (1993): 685.

Jackson, S., A. Weber, T. Hull, et al. "Fecal Incontinence in Women with Urinary Incontinence and Pelvic Organ Prolapse." *Obstetrics and Gynecology* 89 (1997): 423.

Johanson, J., and J. Lafferty. "Epidemiology of Fecal Incontinence: The Silent Affliction." *American Journal of Gastroenterology* 91 (1996): 33.

Nygaard, I., S. Rao, and J. Dawson. "Anal Incontinence After Anal Sphincter Disruption: A 30-Year Retrospective Cohort Study." *Obstetrics and Gynecology* 89 (1997): 896.

Rao, S., K. Welcher, and J. Happel. "Can Biofeedback Therapy Improve Anorectal Function in Fecal Incontinence?" *American Journal of Gastroenterology* 91 (1996): 2360.

Soffer, E., and T. Hull. "Fecal Incontinence: A Practical Approach to Evaluation and Treatment." *American Journal of Gastroenterology* 95 (2000): 1873.

Chapter 12: Sexuality

Berglund, A., M. Eisemann, A. Lalos, et al. "Social Adjustment and Spouse Relationships Among Women with Stress Incontinence Before and After Surgical Treatment." *Social Science and Medicine* 42 (1996): 1537.

Berglund, A., and K. Fugl-Meyer. "Some Sexological Characteristics of Stress Incontinent Women." *Scandinavian Journal of Urology and Nephrology* 30 (1996): 207.

Gordon, D., A. Groutz, T. Sinai, et al. "Sexual Function in Women Attending a Urogynecology Clinic." *International Urogynecology Journal* 10 (1999): 325.

Roe, B., and C. May. "Incontinence and Sexuality: Findings from a Qualitative Perspective." *Journal of Advanced Nursing* 30 (1999): 573.

Weber, A., M. Walters, and M. Piedmonte. "Sexual Function and Vaginal Anatomy in Women Before and After Surgery for Pelvic Organ Prolapse and Urinary Incontinence." *American Journal of Obstetrics and Gynecology* 182 (2000): 1610.

Weber, A., M. Walters, L. Schover, et al. "Sexual Function in Women with Uterovaginal Prolapse and Urinary Incontinence." *Obstetrics and Gynecology* 85 (1995): 483.

American Association of Gynecologic Laparoscopists
13021 East Florence Avenue
Santa Fe Springs, CA 90670-4505
Toll-free number: (800) 554-2245
Fax: (562) 946-9204
E-mail: information@aagl.com
Web site: www.aagl.org

American Urogynecologic Society
2025 M Street NW, Suite 800
Washington, DC 20036
Phone: (202) 367-1167
Fax: (202) 367-2167
E-mail: augs@dc.sba.com
Web site: www.augs.org

Bladder Health Council
American Foundation for Urologic Disease
1128 N. Charles Street
Baltimore, MD 21202
Toll-free number: (800) 242-2383
Fax: (410) 468-1808
E-mail: admin@afud.org
Web site: www.afud.org

The Canadian Continence Foundation
P.O. Box 30, Victoria Branch

Westmount, Quebec
Canada H3Z 2V4
Phone: (514) 488-8379
Toll-free number: (800) 265-9575
Fax: (514) 488-1379
Web site: www.continence-fdn.ca

CONTINENCE RESTORED INC.
407 Strawberry Hill Avenue
Stamford, CT 06902
Day phone: (914) 493-1470
Evening phone: (203) 348-0601

INTERSTITIAL CYSTITIS ASSOCIATION (ICA)
51 Monroe Street, Suite 1402
Rockville, MD 20850
Phone: (301) 610-5300
Toll-free number: (800) 435-7422
Fax: (301) 610-5308
E-mail: ICAmail@ichelp.org
Web site: www.ichelp.org

NATIONAL ASSOCIATION FOR CONTINENCE (NAFC)
P.O. Box 8310
Spartanburg, SC 29305-8310
Phone: (864) 579-7900
Toll-free number: (800) BLADDER [(800) 252-3337]
Fax: (864) 579-7902
E-mail: memberservices@nafc.org
Web site: www.nafc.org

NATIONAL INSTITUTE ON AGING
National Institutes of Health
Building 31, Room 5C27
31 Center Drive, MSC 2292
Bethesda, MD 20892-2292
Phone: (301) 496-1752

Toll-free number: (800) 222-2225
TDD: (800) 222-4225
Fax: (301) 496-1072
Web site: www.nia.nih.gov

NATIONAL KIDNEY AND UROLOGIC DISEASES INFORMATION
CLEARINGHOUSE (NKUDIC)
3 Information Way
Bethesda, MD 20892-3580
Phone: (301) 654-4415
Toll-free number: (800) 891-5390
Fax: (301) 907-8906
E-mail: nkudic@info.niddk.nih.gov
Web site: www.niddk.nih.gov

THE SIMON FOUNDATION FOR CONTINENCE
P.O. Box 835-F
Wilmette, IL 60091
Phone: (847) 864-3913
Toll-free number: (800) 23SIMON [(800) 237-4666]
Fax: (847) 864-9758
Web site: www.simonfoundation.org

Page numbers in *italics* refer to illustrations.

straining during, 40, 69, 183, 219
see also anal incontinence
brain:
 bladder control and, 43–45, 72–73
 injury to, 45
 in rectal control, 218
 rectal control and, 72–73
bulking agents, 222–23
Burch procedure, 124, *125*, 125–26,
 138
 laparoscopic, 126–31, *127*, 148

caffeine, 93, 111
calcium citrate, 164
cancer, 176
 bladder, 25, 65, 157, 158
 radiation therapy for, 28
carbonated beverages, 93, 94, 111
cardinal ligaments, 183
catheters, 53
 placing medicated solutions into
 bladder through, 166–67
 self-catheterization and, 117,
 121–22
cesarean section, 71, 73, 75, 76, 82
 nonmedical reasons to avoid,
 77–78
 as protection against prolapse and
 incontinence, 84–86
 recommendation for more liberal
 approach to, 87–88
 risks and discomfort of, 85
Chamberlain, Pierre, 75
childbirth, 24, 33, 52, 67–88
 anal incontinence and, 78, 81–83,
 217, 218, 222, 225
 baby's size and, 70, 79
 cesarean section in, 71, 73, 75, 76,
 77–78, 82, 84–86, 87–88
 episiotomy in, 73, 83–84, 86–87
 forceps delivery in, 75–76, 82, 87,
 216, 218
 incontinence not inevitable after,
 78–79
 long labor in, 70, 71–73
 natural force of uterine
 contractions in, 73–74, 86

nerves damaged during, 21, 45,
 70–75, 78, 79, 84, 86, 87
 number of babies delivered and,
 70, 79
 occult, or hidden, injuries in, 82,
 84
 pelvic muscles and ligaments
 damaged during, 20, 21, 40,
 70–75, 78, 79, 84, 86, 87, 123,
 175, 180, 181, 183, 202–3, *203*
 preventing incontinence that
 results from, 86–88
 prolapse and, 37–38, 69, 70, 72,
 73, 78, 79–81, 84, 172–74, 175
 reparative surgery after, 81–82, 84
 statistics on incontinence related
 to, 70
chocolate, 93
chronic cystitis, 153
 see also interstitial cystitis
citrus, 93, 111, 164
coffee, 93
cola, 93, 94
colitis, 222
collagen, 22, 40, 45, 69, 212–13
 anal incontinence and, 219, 236
collagen injections, 31, 141–44, *142*,
 148
 success of, 142–43
colonoscopy, 221, 222
colorectal surgeons, 242–43
constipation, 22
contractions:
 in childbirth, 72, 73–74, 86
 Kegel, *see* Kegel contractions
coughing, 60
 leaking during, 18, 19–22, 21, 27,
 37; *see also* stress incontinence
 preventing loss of urine during,
 26, 94, 96
cough stress test, 53
cube pessaries, *194*, 194–95
cystectomy, 170
cystocele, *see* bladder prolapse;
 prolapse
cystocele (anterior) repair, 137, 145,
 146, 202

WILLIAM H. PARKER, M.D.

Dr. William H. Parker is Clinical Professor of Obstetrics and Gynecology at UCLA School of Medicine. He is the former chairman of Obstetrics and Gynecology at Santa Monica–UCLA Medical Center, and is in private practice in Santa Monica.

Dr. Parker is a member of the American Urogynecologic Society and an attending physician at the Pacific Continence Center. He is the author of numerous publications in professional journals on his research findings in the areas of gynecological surgery and laparoscopic surgery. Dr. Parker has also authored several chapters for textbooks standard to the field of gynecologic surgery. Dr. Parker is past president of the American Association of Gynecologic Laparoscopists, and an editor of the *Journal of the American Association of Gynecologic Laparoscopists*. Dr. Parker is a board-certified Fellow of the American College of Obstetricians and Gynecologists.

Dr. Parker is the author of the acclaimed women's health book *A Gynecologist's Second Opinion: The Questions and Answers You Need to Take Care of Your Health*.

Dr. Parker has been selected for both Best Doctors in America and America's Top Doctors.

AMY E. ROSENMAN, M.D.

Dr. Amy E. Rosenman is a co-director of the UCLA Urogynecology Fellowship Program and one of the founders of the Pacific Continence Center in Santa Monica. She is in private practice in Santa Monica, California. Dr. Rosenman is president of the American Urogynecologic Society Foundation and is a published author in the field of urogynecology. She is the former vice-president of the Department of Obstetrics and Gynecology at Saint John's Medical Center and is Assistant Clinical Professor of Obstetrics and Gynecology at the UCLA School of Medicine. Dr. Rosenman is a board-certified Fellow of the American College of Obstetricians and Gynecologists.

In addition, Dr. Rosenman is the medical director of Women's Services at The Center for Healthy Aging. Dr. Rosenman has been selected for both Best Doctors in America and America's Top Doctors.

RACHEL PARKER

In addition to being the mother of three sons, Rachel Parker is a middle-school English teacher with a love for both teaching and writing. Prior to teaching, she worked in public relations and promotion for TV and radio stations. She has also been a community health educator and outpatient mental-health program coordinator at Bellevue Hospital, in New York City.

Dr. Leslie Kaplan is Assistant Clinical Professor, Department of Urology, UCLA School of Medicine, and practices urology in Santa Monica, California.

Dr. Tracy Childs is Clinical Instructor, Department of Surgery, UCLA School of Medicine, and practices colorectal surgery in Santa Monica, California.